Reviews of this book

"I am loving the book. I can so very much relate. I actually laughed out loud at some of the comments your doctors made to you.
I would never go "as easy" on my doc's as you have (in the book)."
Mrs. Karri Stokely, mother of two kids, ex-AIDS patient, Florida, USA

"I devoured your book from start to finish. It is coherent and loaded with information. Writing this book is the work of a Saint. […] I do not know how you found the strength to live through all that. You must truly have a "free spirit", and no doubt this has made you even stronger."
Dennis Dooley, Human Resources Advisor, Ottawa, Canada

"The stark rawness of Maria's journey through years of social and medical prejudice and condescension; the story of her courageous life up to now, is imprinted in her last book *"Goodbye AIDS"*. It is a hymn to the value of human life and to how the efforts of one person may change the world, at least her own world for a start..."
Petros Argyriou, "Zenith" magazine, Thessaloniki, Greece

"Personally, I am persuaded by Maria Papagiannidou. She is a person of blood and flesh who has gone through hell. Her story is both engaging and shocking. But most of all I am persuaded because through her book there comes out a new modus vivendi for the "patients" of AIDS and any other "patients" and, since we are all potential patients, for each one of us: instead of pauperization there is decency, instead of manipulation there is free spirit, instead of the perspective of death, there is a vision for life."
Stopaccius, a blogger in Greece

"Goodbye AIDS! The third part of a trilogy, mature, settled down, without doubts or hesitations. Maria Papagiannidou narrates the age-long adventure she lived up to the point she discovered the Big Truth about AIDS. It is hard to accept that your life was based for 20 years on a Big Lie that was leading you to death. A shocking book."
Erinya, a blogger in Greece

"I have just managed to calm down and stop crying because through your pages I kept reading my own story, with the same thoughts, the same persons (!) but not all the tragic events that happened to you...

Personally, without having done all that so necessary research, I KNOW that things are like that, and the facts that you present them with supporting arguments cause unspeakable joy to me."

Dimitris C. architect, HIV-positive, Greece

Of course you are the lucky person of the story, not because you were "saved" in a sense, but because you went where a lot of us have never been, so that you can tell us now what you saw.

Without exaggerating, I envy you. Fortunately, man possesses imagination and so, like in true theatre, we can live the passion of the other with the same tension, or even maybe with a bigger intensity. I hope I didn't tire you. Personally I feel more rested now.

Charalambos Theodosis, mechanic, Greece

"Bravo to you, bravo, bravo! You are the person who has accumulated all the knowledge a thinking man may need to decide what is better for himself to do, if found "HIV-positive". I won't ever stop thanking you."

Grigoris A. bartender, HIV-positive, Greece

Goodbye AIDS!

Did it ever exist?

by

Maria Papagiannidou-St Pierre

Published by Impact Investigative Media Productions

Author's note
Legal disclaimer

The book that you have chosen to read does not urge anyone to follow a particular therapy for the "medical treatment" of AIDS. It instead deals with the tragic impasse and enormous difficulties of facing a non-existent -- according to the opinion of many experts -- virus. This book reveals, among other things, the surprising absence of reliable evidence for the existence of that virus and for its alleged pathogenicity.

Asserting our freedom of speech and the citizen's rights to information that may contradict official propaganda, I present my personal experience as someone who was considered for a long time to be a "carrier" of the alleged HIV virus and tell of the dramatic course I have travelled from my first positive HIV diagnosis to my recent discoveries that has led to my liberation from the AIDS curse.

Maria Papagiannidou-St Pierre

Acknowledgments

Specials thanks to Penny Xerea and Kim Nickolls for their help with the translation of an early draft of the Greek version, to my husband Gilles Saint-Pierre, and to David Crowe, the president of the Rethinking AIDS international association, as well as to Professor Henry Bauer, who reviewed and edited this book and last, but not least, to my publisher Janine Roberts who did an amazing job giving the book its final touches.

ISBN 978-0-9559177-3-8

English Edition published by Impact Investigative Media Productions
Leonid, Bristol Marina, Hanover Place, Bristol, BS1 6UH. U.K.
Tel. (44) (0)117 925 6818
Email   impactmedia@fearoftheinvisible.com

Impact was founded in 1985 in Australia and moved to the UK in 1990. It has produced investigative films seen on the BBC, WGBH, ABC (Australia) and Channel 4 in the UK, as well as numerous features and investigative works on spiritual, historical, health, environmental and human rights issues. It has also produced films and books on the colonization of Aboriginal Australia.

Cataloguing Information

Health and Fitness: Diseases – AIDS & HIV
Autobiography: Health
Medical: Health Policy

Contents

As a scientist who has studied AIDS for 16 years, I have determined that AIDS has little to do with science and is not even primarily a medical issue. AIDS is a sociological phenomenon held together by fear, creating a kind of medical McCarthyism that has transgressed and collapsed all the rules of science, and imposed a brew of belief and pseudoscience on a vulnerable public.

David W Rasnick, *Blinded by Science,* **Spin, June 1997**

Introduction

When historians look back at our time, they will probably note that the sexual revolution, as a major contribution to the broader movement for human liberation in the 20th century, definitely came to an end in 1984 when the concept of the lethal sexually transmitted 'AIDS' was introduced. Not only did it restrict love, it brought in a disastrous and constant fear. The impact on society was huge.

They will find evidence that after this thousands of people all over the world lost their jobs, their dreams, their human rights. Millions of others who were already living on the edge of death were given the 'coup de grace.' It was called a 'plague,' but this was a massive delusion.

The mass media controlled by a powerful establishment, as experienced in my life, looms large in the background of this story. If we are to truly understand the problems we face, we have to be aware that the restricted information they provide can distort our peception of reality.

It is said that a cure for 'AIDS' cannot be found, but I was 'HIV-positive' for 10 years, had full-blown 'AIDS' for another 12 years and have now become perfectly fine again without any doctor's intervention or medication. My story coincides with the story of 'AIDS' up until now, so I present these stories together to illuminate the true dimensions of 'AIDS'. It is not everlasting or necessary and, to be more precise, it expired before me. How could that happen?

According to the official theory of AIDS that I once believed in, I was doomed to an early death. Actually, I was a dead person for 22 years since there are two kinds of death, the real and the announced one. The latter you carry inside for the rest of your life.

I was researching it as much as possible but for a long while found not a hint that there might be another view of AIDS. However, eventually the fact that I had not met my male heterosexual equivalent during the ten years that I spent going in and out of the hospitals led me to question the sexual transmission dogma and to explore the case deeper on the Internet. I needed an explanation. The unthinkable result was that I came to discover a whole hidden part of the 'AIDS' story that turned the topic upside down. It took me another year to handle the new information and to take an absolutely logical decision: to stop the therapy and 'AIDS' consultations at the age 42, on the 23rd of April 2007. I then began to return to where I was in 1985; to the strong, healthy and optimistic person I was before.

Was it deadly disease that I experienced or a deadly deception? The whole 'AIDS' story has shadowy origins, almost at every step. The normal scientific process was bypassed on the 23rd of April 1984 when the discovery of the 'AIDS' virus was proclaimed to the world weeks before the research data was published and thus before it could be verified by scientists. It was presented as a success of American science that dispelled the fear enshrouding AIDS, mostly due to unreliable epidemiological data gathered from heavy recreational drug users who were far more likely to blame sex than drug usage, since the latter was illegal.

Of course, if a person struggles with drug abuse, chronic heroin, crack addiction or alcoholism, they are also likely to be malnourished. Malnutrition itself is the quickest, most reliable, universal, hundred-percent perfect way of leading to an immune system collapse. No need to invoke a virus.

However, the whole thing was called "AIDS" and attributed to a virus named 'HIV.'

For instance, the first 'AIDS' cases were described, according official reports,[1] in the period October 1980 - May 1981 in 5 young men, all active homosexuals, from 3 different hospitals in Los Angeles, California. Only two of them reported having frequent homosexual contacts with various partners. All 5 reported using inhalant drugs and 1 reported injection drug abuse. The patients did not know each other and had no known common contacts or knowledge of sexual partners who had had similar illnesses.

Nevertheless, a virus was later blamed for their sickness and said to be sexually transmitted.

The 'AIDS' concept then became a greenhouse for complacent scientists who work in an artificial environment, with new criteria, without any real controls, but with much prestige and social status. The syndrome became beneficial to many social groups and, after the launching of the 'AIDS' drugs onto the market, it rose to prominence as an industry with excessive profits.

There is no room for questioning in the 'AIDS' world. Even though about 200 billion dollars has been spent so far on research, the 'HIV/AIDS' theory has failed to produced a cure or a vaccine. The uncritical adherence to the 'HIV' theory continues despite the consequences and despite the fact that more than 2500 professionals (mostly scientists, researchers, doctors and journalists), have shown with solid scientific evidences that this theory is not valid. The latter are discredited a priori as "dissidents" or "denialists" by the 'AIDS' establishment and their questioning is not exposed in the mass media.

However, reliable evidence needs to be present before anyone is told that they are infected with a deadly virus. The patient should also be given a thorough briefing about the subject so he or she can give a proper "informed consent" before taking HIV test that might proclaim one's moribund state, and certainly before beginning treatment for the purported illness.

We do not get that in the case of 'HIV/AIDS'. There is no reliable evidence for the existence of the virus, nor for its pathogenic state, nor its transmission through sexual contact, nor its detection with any test.

I have been considered to be infected with that 'deadly virus' for 24 years,

---

1 CDC MMWR, June 01, 2001 / 50(21);429 First Report of AIDS.
CDC MMWR, June 5, 1981 / 30(21);1-3. Pneumocystis Pneumonia --- Los Angeles

from the first year that the 'HIV' test became available, 1985. What would I have done differently if I knew then what I learned two decades later? Let's examine this together, for I believe I was arbitrarily condemned to an early death sentence, as is now also happening every day to many others.

Personally, I did not receive adequate information about this newly arrived syndrome nor did I have knowledge of the political and economical interests involved, nor the censorship of the critics of the AIDS theory. I only felt the cultural taboo surrounding the disease.

I still have not come to terms with myself after my period of 'AIDS' and it is one of the goals of this book to help me do so. I told my friends for years, reported in my first two books, and repeatedly said, during interviews for the press and TV, that I had first learned in 1995 of my infection with the 'HIV' virus.

That is not exactly the case. The truth is that my forthcoming death was announced to me in 1985 when I was 20 years old. The doctors' advice at that time was not to speak a word of it to others for my own good and I followed their directions. It was costly to me, especially lying to everyone at home, but, believing it was necessary, I could only try to remove it from my mind as best as possible. "You kept it from me an entire year?" my mother asked me painfully when she finally learned the truth in 1996. I was unable to tell her, "I kept it from you eleven years."

When I began my HIVwave.gr web page, wrote my first two books and started giving interviews, I was an 'AIDS' patient taking medication who had already caused much despair to her family. I could not imagine creating any more, for my father had died bitter and so I was determined to hold on to my secret forever.

When I discarded the 'AIDS' medication, I realized that I was not going to die despite all predictions and this enraged me. I was angered for the years of silence, for all that I did unwillingly and for all those ugly things that I could not get rid of – even though I was now doing perfectly fine. Revealing the truth was much harder than quitting the 'AIDS' pills. In my opinion, that is the definition of the so-called plague of the century: lie upon lie, stress upon stress, trap upon trap, much too much for one person to handle. One's mind can be deadly and yet at the same time be emancipating.

The goal of writing this book was also for me to better understand how that universal deception occurred and why it is still alive, though I was lucky enough to escape from its deathly grip before it killed me. My AIDS-patient story alternates with my discoveries at every stage. I hope I can now offer a better "informed consent" to the 'HIV positive' conscripts.

In the first chapter, "What I should not do," I narrate how my life was up until 1985, how perfect everything was and what unsuspecting people I would have to wound by telling them I was bearing the HIV virus. Unless, of course, I kept it a secret. I changed none of my plans and went on to make progress in my studies and in my professional life, although feeling something inside me was broken. In the second chapter, "What was diagnosed for me," I tell how my second positive diagnosis took place in 1995, marking the beginning of my life as an 'AIDS' patient. Apart from again reporting me HIV antibody positive, they detected a "possible" pneumocystis carinii pneumonia infection and low T4 cell count, a condition the doctors assessed meant I now needed 'AIDS' medication. It was a critical decision in which I was not given any room to choose. In the third chapter, "The deleterious side effects of the prescribed therapy", I tell what happpened to me while I took the pills from 1995 until 2007; that is – a series of life-threatening illnesses. It was Dante's Inferno at home and at the hospital.

In the fourth chapter, "How I survived," I tell how I got a breath of fresh air with the creation of my web page, HIVwave.gr, and emails from a Canadian who never found any reliable evidence for 'AIDS' transmission although he was studying biology at McGill University when the discovery of 'HIV' was announced. From the start of our relationship, he showered me with critical information, hoping for my salvation, while a Greek-American scientist, Dr. Maniotis from Chicago, gave me clear instructions on how to cease taking these medications.

In the fifth chapter, "Total supervision by the 'AIDS' establishment", I am overcome by feeling that I am practically criminal and surely dangerous because I no longer accept the classic model of an 'AIDS' patient. I understand how mind-terrorism and taboo mentality are cultivated in the media, by doctors, medical students, activists, each one of us; this being revealed to me by a series of arbitrary events over the final three year period.

In the sixth chapter, "How I regained control of my health," I start building a new life in a world with alternative realities, with new doctors and friends that I could trust.

In the seventh chapter, "How I regained control of my life", I begin posing questions to all I think responsible, speaking more freely in my interviews, meeting willing accomplices along the way, learning of court trials in other countries where the HIV/AIDS concept was questionned, and preparing myself for my return to the world, this time with my own rules.

My long journey proved to be educational. I thank all those I met along the way who somehow managed to widen my horizons. Some are famous and others left anonymous in the text as they requested. Some doctors felt they might damage their career if they were identified as giving me this information, so I have altered their names. I also give only the initials of my 'AIDS' doctors in order to protect them, in the 'AIDS' ambiguous way.

Chapter 1

The Original Sin: What I should not do

I will go far into the past for a while, into my previous life. I learned early on to believe in myself and my parents admired the free spirit I exuded. Along with my independence, I succeeded in all my endeavours. My English, French and piano lessons were sheer entertainment for me. I excelled at piano, although it was my least favourite subject. My parents would say, "What a wise child we have." My brother Stathis was also in this category, "We have two wise children." Within this multifaceted wisdom that I possessed was my love for rock music and I admired Jim Morrison who died aged 27. His death almost seemed conscious. Besides, what's the point of living after 27, I thought. Where would anyone find the zeal to continue doing the same activities in the same high spirit forever?

My mind tossed around these silly ideas as I waited to become an adult. I was accepted into the Philosophy School of Athens, ready to embark on a new voyage. As I discovered the world, I could decide what is worth believing in and what to discard, what I liked and disliked, as my doubts were clarified. Feeling fully armed, I added extras to my curriculum to broaden my horizons. I began taking Italian, drawing, and jazz piano; although I was still not fond of the piano.

I was living at home with dinner ready on the table and someone else to clear up afterwards, leaving me free to explore the world every night. With my two best friends, Vili Kartali and Eva Panagiotakopoulou, we would go out, usually using my house as our base. Eva's mother would sew her dresses and I would sew mine. We mostly tried dressing up and would go out to our usual places which were often two or three different bars in a row.

Nowhere was good enough for us, but we wouldn't lose our temper. We smoked Camel Lights. Smokers we were not, but under the strong lights and loud megaphones, a cigarette would help overcome the lack of discussion.

During my second year at university I met my first true love. The School of Philosophy was then located in the School of Law building on Solonos Street, and was experiencing a shortage of men. To be exact, there were 2 or 3 men for 500 women. Naturally I looked elsewhere for someone to strike my fancy. The student body of the neighbourhood did not impress me as much as did one man who frequented the bar Enallax in the Exarheia district.

The "stranger" of Enallax was much older, 31. He had a Pharmacist's degree from Italy, he was well traveled, read foreign fiction and was writing his own book. He even danced differently, with strange movements. At some point, I saw his cologne at home, Van Kleef & Arpels. The first gift he had for me was the little book of Arthur Schnitzler *"Night Games"* (1926), the loveliest novel I had ever read. Many of my fellow students would gather in the evening at the same bar but I would go to see Dimitri and talk. The world he so eloquently spoke of was unknown to me. I was astonished.

Would he be the man of my destiny? Our relationship was the best two years of my life up to then. I got through my courses singing. Dimitri had told me of his drug experiences in Italy, but this belonged to his past. My desire to hear him speak was insatiable, I was in love. I gave no relevance to the drugs as they had no part in our daily lives. Every night we would go to another tavern in Exarheia for dinner, to another bar for music, to his place for love.

Drugs I never tried, either before Dimitri or after, I felt no need for them. At home we were happy anyway. "I haven't ever seen a family like yours, not having any problem", a lady friend of my brother had once said. "Your only worry is if the cat doesn't empty its bowl." In the meantime, my mind was constantly searching for new opportunities. Vili and I opted to go on an InterRail trip across Europe with one month unlimited train rides for people 20-25 years old. We were 20 and began our excursion equipped with steak sandwiches made by Vili's mother. It was 30 days of sleeping on the train and three stops in between for rest, in Stockholm, Paris and Manchester.

Upon returning to Athens we were exhausted, but filled with satisfaction. Vili reunited with her soul mate Giorgos and I with an enthused Dimitri. Until everything changed within the blink of an eye. One night I saw him intoxicated, actually high. "Someone offered me some stuff for one time use," he told me. I did not run, thinking I could reason with him. He was so intelligent, how could he do such a thing? He was abusing heroin again, I didn't need long to work this out for he admitted it. He said he would stop but it was too late. It caused me great pain that I could do nothing to help him.

The worst part was his phone call revealing that he had been found "HIV positive." I have tried to recall how things transpired at the time, unable to speak of it until now. I still do not know how I managed to keep my secret for so long, finding out that I too was HIV positive shortly after Dimitri, in the August of 1985. He sent me this letter soon afterwards:

It is a peculiar feeling, sweet heart. I first felt it when I was told that there was a problem. "You have been infected with the virus." Actually, it is not one feeling, it is many together. Bitterness, sadness, frustration, fear, fear again, pain, paranoia, desolation and desolation times ten and I do not know what else.

This is the last letter I will send you, undated, yet with many tears and one wish. One wish which I honestly want to come true. Something I have been wishing for 15 days now. If there is a god, dammit (I never asked for one to exist), not knowing what else to say, as long as you have nothing they can tell me I have 15 days to live. Believe me, little one, I want nothing else from life, only that you are well and know that this Dimitri holds you in greater esteem than himself. My mind thinks of nothing but you these days. That face that I love so much is the one I have harmed. I do not want you to feel hatred towards me, it was not my mistake. I want you to be well and if this is an unpleasant chapter in your life then I want you to turn the page, or rather burn it. I just hope you are well. Forgive me if I have done something that could hurt you. I will love you forever, Dimitri.

Feel hatred? It was more like bewilderment mixed with horror. My first test results were negative but I had to repeat the test three weeks later, and so was unable to escape the bad news. I felt the earth moving under my feet, even though I was unable to conceive the meaning of it for me. Would I meet the fate of all those who perished within a few months? Strange, I was still feeling good. It was hard to believe that I was going to die. It' s not easy to prepare for death when you are 20 and healthy, I had to work on it thoroughly.

The next day was my name day celebration and everyone was joyous for me. I cannot forget the only thought that was going through my brain. It was how long could I fool everybody? When the time came, I would hurt them more than they could ever expect. Perhaps there was a way to avoid it? As Dimitri thought only of me, I thought only of my mother, father and brother. The news would devastate them. "How soon will treatment be available?" I asked the doctor who gave me my test results. "It is going to be a while." "How long?" "Perhaps ten years, maybe more." In another doctor's office, in another building on another floor, I remember how Dr. G.P., the AIDS director at the time, meticulously perused my arms searching for signs of drug use. He was disgruntled again that he had found no trace of this. "You don't have to do anything for now", he said. 'The virus will not be activated for a while and is spread through sexual contact. So, use condoms during sex and do not tell anybody, not even your family". I left with a small wish to have no need for him any time soon and the reality is, I never saw him again.

Dimitri was shaken when I revealed to him my diagnosis. We barely discussed the situation. The news at the time was that the virus had made its way to Italy from America and had arrived on our shores in the summer of 1985, as if it had come with luggage or with a specific load of drugs that Dimitri's circle of friends were taking. I became officially one of the first recipients of that new virus in Greece.

I did not blame him, for I was not preoccupied with pointing fingers. It was inconceivable what would take place from here on and what burned inside me: that I would have the next ten years to contemplate and conceal the truth was no comfort. I had been more or less immobilized. Even if I divulged the truth, no one could help me, I would only succeed in saddening the lives of those around me. There are no words of consolation here, the effort is futile.

"I want you to promise we will reveal nothing. We'll forget it," I requested Vili and Eva that first week. We had a consensus. Besides. there was a degree to finish and post-graduate studies to begin. One matter was pending, a visit to Evangelismos Hospital for an immune system test that involved a blood examination. Vili accompanied me and for the first time I witnessed nurses approaching with caution, as if I had grown scales. They were completely cloaked and wore nylon masks. My friend felt ashamed for their behaviour. Fortunately, I happened to have a 1,400 T4 or CD4 count, which pleased them. They even managed to crack a smile.

I had no intention of returning to that place without a reason and certainly not with a friend or acquaintance. Upon leaving I made the decision to continue to live normally and to wait patiently for a treatment to be found. What disheartened me the most was the inability to have a long-term relationship. Dimitri and I parted yet remained close friends, I completed my degree with honours and began preparing for a Master's degree in London. Eva and I became inseparable twins during our last year at the university. In the end she stayed on in England after her post-graduate studies and is still there, a lecturer in Archaeology at the University of Edinburgh.

Vili and I departed for London in September of 1987. Intense studying was the rule for all of us and our stamina inexhaustible. I received my Master's Degree with Distinction at the end of the year, possibly a reaction to my invisible illness. I even had a three-day relationship with a French student, wanting to try out the doctor's advice about using protection, something I would not repeat often, since it felt uncomely and obligatory to me.

I returned to Athens in August of 1988. In September I began a journalism apprenticeship at the newspaper "*To Vima*,"[2] and in January of 1989 I was put on their payroll. For some reason I've always completed tasks with ease since childhood and take joy in this. My new program at work proved no different. I participated eagerly and realized surprisingly that I was always myself.

While at the newspaper I learnt of a fact that seemed like a saving grace: the virus could only be spread through blood and sperm. I had not been told this earlier, what an oversight! So I cannot spread it. It was a drop in the ocean, yet comforted me. Why hadn't doctor G.P. told me this? Maybe he hadn't known this in 1985, and I wouldn't go to ask him anything again. I tried some casual or almost free relationships but they seemed to be so meaningless since I would probably soon become sick and die. I dropped them as quickly as possible and turned back to myself. I could participate in anything else joyfully. My illness was buried deep inside me and I wanted to delight undisturbed in the praises of my superiors and co-workers. The thought "How much will I disappoint them too in time," often came to me.

Even worse, at home when the television showed AIDS patients dying helplessly, my father would say, "Fortunately we do not have such problems at home" and change the channel, unable to handle the suffering. I wanted to drop off the face of the earth but instead went out as often as possible, at least when Eva came to visit from England. We then had our most glorious evening outings at the club "Koukos" in Athens.

---

2   *To Vima* is a high profile newspaper in Greece, published daily except on Mondays, and its flagship is the Sunday edition.

I rented a house in the historical Plaka[3] district, wanting to be alone and unseen. I could begin writing an article at three in the morning and have it ready for work by noon. I would walk to the old "Vima" offices in Karytsi Square, discuss the article with the head editor, return home to sleep until the evening and plan my next excursion. When Eva was away, I would sometimes go out alone, drive around singing my favourite songs until reaching my club destination where I would hang out with the DJ who would welcome my presence even without Eva. They were pointless efforts, but at least filled my time. "So we hear you party every night," I was told at work. They were always proud of me. Dimitri did not stop sending letters to my home. We would see each other occasionally but those were awkward moments. I recently found a letter from him in 1989 and I've included it to show what a man he was and what intuition he possessed:

> Four years have passed since we first met. Four years of a beautiful and ugly relationship marked surreptitiously and indecently from one event. I do not wish to characterize it differently. No matter what I say or write to you, I should be the one ashamed to confront you and not have the audacity to request a rendezvous, to go to dinner or even worse to make love to you. I want you to believe me, this is how I have been feeling, especially lately. There are times when you ask what is wrong and what I am thinking when I am not speaking or laughing. What is on my mind? Always the same thing. I want to tell you that I love and desire you yet I cannot utter the words upon seeing you. I wish I could be different each time we meet. This is how I am, how I have learned to be, how I truthfully feel about you because I love you, want you and miss you. I am impudent even to write such nonsense, you will probably say, however it is not easy to stop. You cannot fathom how much I wish everything was different or at least that one thing had not occurred. You would be the great love of my life forever. It is not like it was not that way anyhow, at least some time ago. Yet every time I face you, I find you do not have my feelings of guilt. Each time I see you, I become schizophrenic, two sides wrestling inside me with no champion. I think of the game tic tac toe in this circumstance. Did you ever play it when you were young? It is a very insipid game where no one wins. It is comparable to my incorrigible psychological state every time I think of you. Love and longing on the one hand, euphoria in other words, and revulsion for myself on the other.
>
> I often dream, unable to do otherwise, of past times and seasons and how we could have been. It is at that moment I begin to weep and get infuriated wanting to ram my head into the wall while wishing I could

---

3   The Plaka in Athens is in the shadow of the Acropolis, like a village within the city, a popular neighborhood.

just call you and say 1000 and more lovely things, sweet and unimportant. Yet I will never do it, I remain dreaming....

Return to the present now, as I hold the letter in my hand: "Surreptitiously and indecently," is how he described what appeared in our lives. I had the same feeling without being able to explain it. Dimitri died much later from AIDS, I was told, while taking anti-HIV therapy. I assumed for years that the HIV virus had killed him; that is, until "X", a friend who wished to remain anonymous, wrote to me:

> The HIV virus has never been isolated anywhere. If someone has doubts they can quite easily confirm this truth without futile refutations. One merely needs to request the original scientific publication. Normally it would be easily accessible from the Department of Health or the universities could provide the related scientific publication, if it exists. In Germany, Austria, Italy and elsewhere this has not been proved possible despite 12 continuous years of questions posed to those in authority from citizens and scientists alike; because they never existed.

It seems inconceivable today that the virus has never been isolated (so long have they been fooling us?) but we did not doubt it, even in 1985, when the bomb blew up in our midst, only one year after the cause of AIDS was announced by the USA's Secretary of Health Margaret Heckler in an international Press Conference. Her statement referred to HIV being the 'possible cause' of AIDS but curiously the word 'possible' was omitted from the subsequent press reports. The general feeling was that it must be certain as no objections were voiced. The Australian professor Hiram Caton wrote ten years later in his book *The AIDS Mirage*[4]:

> The journalists reporting this event didn't notice the telltale signs that there was something fishy about the occasion. An obvious anomaly was that the announcement was made prior to publication of the articles presenting the evidence. A firm rule of scientific publication bans this practice. It hobbles the critical reception because scientists cannot comment on research that they haven't seen. [...]
>
> As it happened, there were quite a few scientists who gave Gallo's claims little credence. But their voices were not heard because the journalists didn't search for critical comments. And in a very short time the orthodoxy was so entrenched that critical views seemed aberrant, even "loony."

The journalists could have corrected the omission when claims such as Hiram Caton's began to surface in 1995. Strangely, that never happened. They

---

4   Hiram Caton, <u>The AIDS Mirage, 1995</u> chapter 6 "Junk Science Goes Belly-Up"

neglected for some reason to do their basic task which is to examine their source of information. However, I did not know this at the time. It is possible that the HIV virus never existed and that I was never infected with anything.

Thus my mistake was not falling in love with someone who didn't follow the conventions. It was something else, not quite tangible. Perhaps it was believing all I was told by the "scientific" experts on the subject? I could not imagine that those experts really did not know and could have been misled.

Chapter 2

Retribution: What was diagnosed for me

The period after 1985:

For nine years after the first detection of the virus supposedly in my blood, everything was under control. No suspicions at home and, in order to be certain, I played my role ever more convincingly. Only my father would sometimes say, "The time has come for you to find a man in your life." I acted like I did not understand at first, then rented the house in Plaka simply to avoid hearing it. In 1990, with Gianni Pretenteri as head editor, the newspaper *To Vima* added a section called "New Times". I took over the two central pages discussing trends in the book market, and for about five continuous years I produced good articles, gaining a respectable reputation at the newspaper and in the world of publishing. All this gave me satisfaction and kept me alive. In the meantime, I made many trips as a result of professional invitations to Venice, Yugoslavia, Egypt, New York, Washington and Turkey.

I became melancholic when in other cities, as I thought about the lovely places I would never be able to enjoy with a partner. This was most intense in Montenegro during an evening of welcoming festivities before Yugoslavia split apart. We were the formal guests of the State Department of the country and three gypsies with violins stood in front of our table with drunken smiles. As I saw them approaching I stood up. They began playing divine melodies and singing words of love I did not understand but I wanted to cry. Will these people ever have AIDS? I doubt it. What mistake had I made? I only fell in love. Why could I not be a gypsy? Then a desire came over me – I wanted to fall in love with the first man to cross my path. But then I remembered that was forbidden for me. The frustration did not leave me for the remainder of the trip.

Back in Athens the same year, 1990, I began having some strange health ailments, the first being a herpes zoster outbreak on my thorax which disappeared quickly and then, in 1992, a rash on my face like severe acne. It was staphylococcus which required many visits to the dermatologist. It was the first time a doctor became essential to my life.

A slight hope occurred when my brother opened an Internet account at home, one of the first in Greece. I began searching there for more information on AIDS, even though Google search did not exist then. However, the few web pages that I found were not really helpful at all.

I hesitantly put the dating game back in my life but it just resulted in two or three short relationships soon after. Then, in 1993, a relationship slipped out of my control and began developing into something serious. I became panic stricken, because he wanted to marry me.

Around 1994 my output at work began to decrease, any evening outings were at a minimum, as were just about everything else I tried to do. During a summer holiday with my partner of that time, Niko Vrahno, the sight of any hill would make me walk in the opposite direction. "Let's take another road," I would hear myself saying, taking the lead. Later on in Athens, the weight of my head seemed unbearable as I struggled to keep my eyes on my computer screen. Had AIDS come knocking on my door? I'd have to collapse without breathing a word. I would be carried on a stretcher, dying quickly to end it all. I was prepared for this scenario, I saw it approaching. Had I instigated this? Was I at fault? It all transpired in a manner similar to what I expected. During Easter of 1995 I had an unrelenting fever and Niko took me first to the doctor of the EODEAP[5] and then to the Athens Medical Center as it was covered by the insurance I received from the Journalists' Union. I endured a week of examinations, all of which had negative results, but they could not find the cause of my illness. The doctors would come in and out, studying me nervously and encouraging me to be patient. They had no other alternatives.

Finally I suggested they perform an AIDS test. The doctors looked upon me with gratitude. Good thinking! They retreated and asked for a nurse to take a blood sample.

In the days that ensued two doctors and a nurse reappeared dressed as astronauts. They stood in a row protected by their masks and revealed the positive results of the test. I was then escorted to the proper unit. The work of those doctors was completed, having nothing else to contribute.

I was apparently infected by the HIV virus, which means special care. They only inquired as to which hospital would I prefer to be sent to, the Laiko or Evangelismo, for these had special units for people with my illness. To avoid any potential encounters with acquaintances at Evangelismo I chose the Laiko. Fortunately my mother was away from Athens at the time. She was working as a high-school principal on the island of Evia. My father, a former high-school principal himself, had retired early owing to heart problems, but he always stayed uninvolved with my personal life.

At the Laiko Hospital, the doctors actually had some expertise with AIDS. First, they dressed as civilians, not spacemen, and were not frightened. This was very comforting. However, there was an impenetrable wall of silence around the decisions made for my treatment. The doctors seemed to be part of a secret society that only the initiated could join. I had AIDS and I had to trust them if I wanted to survive. Also, they emphasized that it was best not to say anything to anybody.

After I recovered from the fever, Niko and I left the hospital, returned home and attempted to put our thoughts in order. Niko was the one thunderstruck this time and, curiously, he reacted in the same fashion as I had in 1985. He was devastated and distressed yet did not blame me for one second. There was one difference, though. He tested negative for the antibodies. He repeated the test

---

5   EDOEAP, the Health and Pension Association of Journalists

twice more and was still negative. "Do not waste your time, the virus cannot be transmitted from a woman to a man, I have read it," I told him. Niko stayed with me for some time despite the predicament becoming unbearable for him.

My good doctors said I had reached the final stage of AIDS. I had now been infected for about ten years and my T4 cell count had dropped to 26 – according to which I should have already died. My delayed visit to the doctors had contributed, they said, to the fatal progression of the disease. They understood everything! I should have even apologized in the end. They could only offer me a short extension of my life with the drug AZT and I thanked them. I asked for a leave of absence from the newspaper for a month and a half to contemplate what to do.

Back home my family was still unaware. At work the word spread almost immediately through the journalist association EDOEAP. I am not certain if it was morally permitted to disclose it, but in the long run it was favourable. I had instigated it by requesting such a long leave of absence and soon I was called by the secretary to Stavros Psyharis, the director of the newspaper, asking me to come to his office when I could. I went the following day and he knew. He asked me nothing and only commented that I look great now, not to worry, I had the leeway to not come to work as long as I needed and would still be paid my salary. I did not return before the entire leave had finished as I truly needed time to recover from the last announcement at Laiko Hospital. I eventually returned to the office to gather all the support I needed. At home, I could keep it a secret indefinitely. Things were not quite so ugly after all, I had made a complete recovery.

Return to the present:

What exactly had been diagnosed that convinced the doctors that I had developed AIDS? My doctors said it was my low T4 cell count, the pneumocystis carini pneumonia and the new positive HIV test – they had no idea that I had tested postitive over ten years earlier. It made sense to me.

At that time, I felt certain about the information I was acquiring about the disease. I was being educated by a doctor and university professor, T.K., while everything I read on the Internet seemed to describe my situation. I had done an ELISA test in 1985 and again in 1995 with the blood sample sent by the Athens Medical Center to the proper unit. Afterwards, the Western Blot test had confirmed the results with the blood sample from the Laiko Hospital, again at the proper unit. These were the tests used for AIDS so I had taken the right steps.

Yet, I had not been informed by anyone in 1985 nor in 1995 that on the boxes in which these tests came there were labels with inscriptions that told of the doubts of the manufacturers about the validity of their own tests. It is possible that even the doctors were unaware of this. The pharmaceutical companies, however, know how to protect themselves from lawsuits. I saw it once in the "*The Other Side of AIDS,*" a film of Robin Scovill (2004) and again recently, in an interview given by a professor at the University of Chicago, Dr. Maniotis, to our correspondent in Washington, Lambros Papantoniou. It was published in November of 2007 in Athens in the weekly independent newspaper

"Friday + 13" with the heading "AIDS: A Worldwide Scandal." This is from that interview:

> The makers of the test kits used to measure "HIV," or progression to "AIDS", are themselves aware of these issues, because they all claim their ELISA, Western Blot and PCR-based kits can't really detect the "HIV" virus.

> For example, Abbott Laboratory's ELISA HIV test kit package insert says that ELISA testing alone cannot be used to diagnose AIDS.

> Perhaps the most important statement on Abbott's insert says that, "at present, there is no recognized standard for establishing the presence or absence of HIV antibody in human blood."

> Epitope's Western Blot test kit insert says, "do not use this kit as the sole basis for diagnosing HIV infection."

> Roche's PCR amplicor HIV monitor test says that it is not intended to be used as a screening test for HIV, nor as a diagnostic test to confirm HIV infection.

> The NucliSens HIV assay says that it is not intended to be used as a screening test for HIV, nor used as as diagnostic test to confirm the presence of HIV-1 infection.

> COBAS AmpliScreen HIV-1 test says that it is not intended for use as an aid in diagnosis.

> The Cambridge Biotech's HIV Western Blot Kit insert says that the clinical implications of antibodies to HIV in an asymptomatic person are "not known." This caveat on the package insert is actually a printed concession that it is not known whether HIV is the cause of AIDS. It's right there – in the HIV test kit itself.

> We are constantly being told by the media and government that the clinical significance of the presence of the antibodies means that you are going to die of AIDS eventually. How can they give drugs to millions on other continents or to infants, or to anyone else, without knowing what the clinical significance of testing positive is? What is its purpose then? If it isn't a screening or diagnostic test, then what kind of test is it? A lie detector to see if you've been sleeping around?

The manufacturers' inserts in the test kits have continually changed from 1984 until now. The manufacturers [6] have included more and more doubts in the wording in order to be absolved from any responsibility in case they are obliged to defend themselves. It is almost as if they have sensed that some people have caught on and are attempting to maneuvre more adroitly. From 1984 the legal statement included with the ELISA HIV test was that "AIDS is caused by HIV." In November 2002 a new insert began to appear "AIDS: AIDS–related-complex and pre-AIDS are THOUGHT TO BE CAUSED by

---

6 From Alive & Well emailer, November 13, 2003 "Hidden Facts of HIV Tests: What's in the Fine Print", by Christine Maggiore.
http://www.aliveandwell.org/html/questioning/hidden_facts.html, accessed Dec. 27, 2008.

HIV" and now we have the still weaker statement that "published data indicate a strong correlation between AIDS and a retrovirus called HIV." This last quote is found in the package insert for a new ELISA test (Vironostika HIV-1 Plus O Microelisa System) approved by the FDA in June 2003.

So, what is the meaning of a positive 'HIV' test result? The wonderful scientist and microbiologist Angelos Sicilian, whom I would meet later, attempted to clarify this. I will use this name for him in this book, since he has asked to remain anonymous, fearing the risks for his professional career from the 'AIDS' establishment. He wrote to me:

> To my knowledge, for the first time in epidemiological history a medical paradox has been introduced. In some parts of the world there is an increase of incidence while in others a decrease. In particular; Africa and the United States report a rise while in Europe the number of cases has declined. This epidemiological paradox is likely due to the existence of different diagnostic criteria.
>
> In other words, the shuffling of diagnostic results in Europe is more humane than in the countries where there is a decline in humanity, as in the United States, where the diagnoses continue to increase. The same is occurring in Africa, except in South Africa where president Thabo Mbeki has raised his stature by opposing the doubtful conjectures that have proved very profitable and evidently been transformed into 'certainties.' However, he is paying a significant political cost for his stand.
>
> That is all for the so-called ELISA HIV 1-2 test. Now as far as the Western Blot test is concerned, the AIDS specialists have exalted its diagnosis to gold standards. It is enough to read a report by Eleni Papadopoulos-Eleopoulos* from Australia to understand that a fortune teller would have the same success at deciphering the complicated patterns of such an uncertain test. (*Eleni-Papadopulos-Eleopulos, Valendar F. Turner and John M. Papadimitriou Bio/Technology Vol.11 June 1993 Is a Positive Western Blot Proof of HIV Infection?) It is about a test whose specifications have not been established anywhere using a precise standard. The curious and somewhat suspicious part is that this test only takes place at certain laboratories, is restricted and not even taught in public laboratories.

In the past few years, a US$50,000 reward has been on offer for locating any study published in a peer-reviewed medical journal that validates any HIV test by finding and isolating HIV in fresh tissue samples taken from the person testing positive.[7] As long as no winner does emerge to claim this reward, how illogical is it to suggest that we should stop doing those tests? And, of course, to

---

7 From Christine Maggiore's organization "Alive and Well AIDS Alternative" in Los Angeles http://www.aliveandwell.org/html/award.html (accessed December 27, 2008).

discontinue treatments for a virus that is undetectable?

One question remains. What causes the ensuing deadly AIDS if not the HIV virus? Part of the answer has been provided by a witness of the events during the period when the syndrome first appeared, a specialist in AIDS medication and researcher of protease inhibitors, David Rasnick: 'AIDS in the 1980's was primarily a result of the recreational drug epidemic in the United States and in Europe. However, it shifted considerably in the 1990's. In the 1990's at least half of all new AIDS cases, maybe even 60% now, are the direct result of the antiretroviral therapies themselves.'

Not only were many of the side effects of the first anti-retroviral therapy similar to those ascribed to AIDS, it was estimated that in the first decade of AZT, 1987-1997, more Americans died from them than were killed in the Vietnam war, almost 300.000 young men.

However, when offered the anti-retroviral medication in 1995, I was not aware of the warnings that had already been presented in the book *THE AIDS WAR: Propaganda, Profiteering and Genocide from the Medical-Industrial Complex*, published in 1993 by John Lauritsen[8].

> A PWA [Person With Aids] will not survive unless he maintains independence from doctors. The bitter reality is that almost all doctors treating AIDS patients are prescribing nucleoside analogues, thus ensuring a fatal outcome

Due to my innocence I agreed to start the drugs.

---

8   John Lauritsen, *THE AIDS WAR: Propaganda, Profiteering and Genocide from the Medical-Industrial Complex* Asklepios, 1993 (p. 215).

Chapter 3

Inferno: The deleterious side effects of the prescribed therapy

Back to 1995.

I began taking AZT as prescribed, the only medication for AIDS then available in Greece. But then I had second thoughts. I felt I still had time to decide on another course since I was feeling good again. I discovered through an Internet search that my only alternative was a healthy diet consisting of roots and plant extracts in a retreat for AIDS patients on a Spanish island. Wanting to disappear, I found the idea enticing. After discussing that opportunity with Anna Vlavianou, a journalist colleague, she requested for me a financial boost of 1,000,000 drachmas (about 3,000 Euros) from Stavros Psixaris, the editing manager of our newspaper to cover the costs of the trip, and he agreed.

But when I told Dr. Kordosi about my decision, he replied, "Without medication you have about ten days left." Shaken, I thanked him for rescuing me from charlatans and continued taking AZT. It seemed like a mild pill, I was not experiencing any side-effects yet. I was given the pills in a generic bottle, with a 'Retrovir' (commercial name of AZT) label that had no warnings. "Soon the scientists will discover a miraculous cure and this will be over before anyone finds out", I thought, "before the summer ends, everything will be different".

I still could not tolerate the idea of how much pain my AIDS diagnosis would cause my family. I had not even told my brother. After repeated requests, my dear doctor agreed to book an appointment at a hospital in London for re-examination. A friend from the newspaper, Kosmas Vidos, offered to accompany me and we went to St. George's Hospital in November of 1995. My results were positive again and my diagnosis the same. "You have about 4 years left at best." So I have gained an extension due to the AZT, I thought. Who knows what else will be found by the scientists in such a period of time! I proceeded to go on a shopping spree in London. I was given a death sentence, but still felt fine. I had lost control of my life though, it was clear; and I only had to think how I will escape attention of the others, how I will fool my family and for how long, how I will come back from London as if it was an entertainment trip. But why had not any other symptom appeared yet besides that pneumonia? I would now ask myself how it could be possible for such a catastrophe to be happening, and me to be still alive. I was observing everything in astonishment from the outside looking in.

The tide would not take long to turn. AIDS or AZT, for I had heard the worst of both, would soon show their true faces. By Christmas my condition had seriously worsened. I had a fever of 40C (104 Fahrenheit) while at home with my brother and had to tell him the truth. He was devastated. He embraced me strongly while mumbling, "What are you telling me now?" He was unable to believe what I had just told him. I was hardly hearing his voice, there was no time to lose, he rang the emergency unit and we were soon taken to the hospital. I awoke the following morning to find my mother in front of me, looking me tenderly in the eyes. "It's not your fault," she said with all her love. "You had one misfortune in your life and this is it. We'll overcome it." What is she saying, I thought in despair. Mothers are unbelievable!

At some point I was released from the hospital – rooms were desperately needed, only emergencies could be accommodated. I was soon to return due to severe anaemia. An acknowledged side-effect of AZT, as I now know, but did not know then.

The agonizing blood transfusions started, we needed a constant supply and each time we had to wait endlessly for them to locate my blood type. I was in and out of consciousness and do not remember how long I stayed there nor how many transfusions I was given. When all that came to an end I was released from the hospital and driven home to continue my therapy. Soon, my nervous disorder would become so serious that tingling would not let me rest at all, night or day. I needed a bucket of cold water underneath my blankets to wet my feet which felt like they were on fire, a side effect of drugs known as peripheral neuropathy. This was the most intense this symptom would ever be. During this period, I remember also having oral thrush. My tongue hurt so much I was unable to rest it on my teeth. I could not eat, speak or drink water. My only consolation was Xylocaine, a syrup that numbed my mouth. "Take Xylocaine in moderation," I was told by the hospital dentist. "It is my only pleasure," I jotted on my notepad that I kept in my pocket in order to communicate. This was also the most intense thrush I would ever have. All these symptoms poured down on me like a hurricane. There was no time even to weep.

When the wooden mouth finally passed, I still could not eat due to my anemia and low blood count. My mother attempted to raise it by putting everything in the blender, fruits, vegetables, even meat. Yet I was unable to touch any of it. Finally, I was given medication for an unrelated illness which increased my appetite as a side-effect. This did the job. Within one month I was fat from the waist up. My mother's joy was indescribable. She saw that we could have results through our efforts. I felt our efforts pointless, but wouldn't say so. My blood count remained low as well as my stamina. "This is how you should have always been, a little on the plumper side," my mother would say to break the silence.

Soon afterwards, in September of 1996 I was diagnosed with cytomegalovirus of the eyes which would have blinded me had a new strew of pills not been discovered. It was twelve pills per day which at least had recently replaced the shots as treatment for this condition. I began contemplating blindness along with everything else. I had to prepare myself for the possibility since there was no certainty with the treatment. We would have to wait and see. Surely I was once again fortunate for the recent discovery of this new medication.

"Just discovered", I would hear each time I began a new treatment. I would be the first guinea pig and apparently the only survivor at the end. I was truly lucky, being saved in the nick of time. Many whom I roomed with, or who were my neighbours in the hospital, died that summer. Out of them, I was the only one left alive in September 1996 when the protease inhibitor drugs appeared on the market. So, the twelve pill treatment for cytomegalovirus was combined for me with my first cocktail medication of Norvir, 3TC and Hivid. I was now taking 23 pills daily and this powerful combination got me back on my feet (however, perhaps stopping AZT was all that was required). I even managed to baptize the firstborn son of Vili. She insisted that we had agreed on my becoming the godmother. It was Easter of 1997 and, strangely, that day I felt beautiful.

The treatment for cytomegalovirus ceased after two years. I had escaped blindness. I now had to make weekly visits to the hospital for a special IV that would neutralize some dangerous side-effect from my treatment. My mother would accompany me and support me through the corridors and check-in. "I should be supporting you mom, not the opposite," I would tell her each time I leaned on her. "It doesn't matter sweetie, it's only temporary," she would respond as we got in the car. She would leave me waiting on a bench in front of the hospital and then go search for parking on some street in the Goudi neighbourhood. I would then see her rushing towards me to pick me up and continue inside for that despicable IV. Each time I saw her approaching, tranquillity would overcome me for a bit. I needed no one, only wanting my mother. With her I felt protected from all forms of evil, she was my shield. We would enter the out-patients room and wait for the nurses to come.

I would wake up at 7 o'clock in the morning to get this over with. The nurses would begin their rounds at the opposite end of the corridor, even though they had seen us waiting for one IV only. The treatment room for HIV was located in the same wing as Gynaecology and Otorhinolaryngology so as not to draw any attention and traumatize the other patients. Naturally the nurses recognized us from afar each time we arrived. I wanted it known that I was no longer hospitalized. "Why am I taken last every time?" I snapped at the nurse when she came after one hour. "Do you think the hospital functions for you only? We have many jobs to do here," she replied. "And I'm one of those jobs," I continued with the same tone and managed to irritate her just as she searched for a vein to poke. The vein search had become the most difficult task for the hospital staff. In both arms my veins had either broken or clotted. One nurse would fail, another would make an attempt, also failing. I sat silently at this point, while my mother would nervously search for the one kind and patient nurse who had succeeded several times. It was unknown each time how long this would take, yet it had to be completed every time.

The torture would then begin. Once the IV was in, my stomach would ache during the 3-4 hours it would take for the bottle above my head to finish, drop by drop. "You should let the IV drop more slowly to avoid upsetting your stomach," each nurse would say passing by my room. Any slower, the IV would take ten hours. I would attempt to see how quickly I could administer the flow. I held the control in my hand. My mother was always by my side to console me. "Have patience, see how nice it is here just the two of us. They're all gone. What's the hurry to go home. What do you have to do there?" I did not answer being lost in thought. "Look at what a mom I have. I've embittered her so much. I'm an idiot, stupid, worthless, laughable." "You have come 165 times," I was told by the secretary at the reception desk. I prayed for the day that I would never see her again. However, the next stage was only that my IV changed from once per week to once every two weeks. I cannot recall when I stopped those visits, probably when I changed treatment.

I was also going to the newspaper, feeling as good as a normal person for a while. Nikos Bakounakis, leading the Books section during my period of severe side-effects and little hope, seemed to still count on me. I liked that, and wanted to prove him right. I wouldn't stay too long there, yet the job got done. He would welcome my new suggestions for articles, so I could withdraw with a victorious smile to work on them at home. Where did I find the new ideas since I was constantly stuck in bed, nobody asked, they all seemed happy to see me around. Thanks to my good friend Kostas Voukelatos, publisher of `Ichneutis` magazine and founder of book statistics in Greece, I wouldn't be left for a single day without a long, delightful, informative phone call. "Don't give up now", he would say to me if I sounded frustrated and weak. "I have a good topic for you. You will love it". If I was not able to go out, he would send me what I needed by mail.

Apart from that, I was fully occupied just taking the pills on time. We had to store the Norvir in the refrigerator and even had an ice cooler in the freezer just in case I needed to take the pills with me when going out. I would sneak to the refrigerator like some thief and swallow three giant Norvir pills three times per day, and my mother would bring me the rest – together with antibiotics, not to be forgotten. At least my father never asked about those bottles in the refrigerator. But the "occasional" infections "due to the virus" would not let me rest at all. New antibiotics would each time be prescribed together with the AIDS medication, causing more thrush as a side effect. This left me in a constant state of emergency, no matter how much I watched out.

Lipodystrophy, a side effect of the AIDS medication, continued to distort my appearance. I became big from the waist up, lean on the legs and bottom. Knowing I had no choice, I would see this and try to overlook it. Soon I would die after all. I had been baptised into the religion of AIDS since 1996, when my treatment program required that I consume those 23 pills daily. A metamorphosis took place over the years. One changes into a monk or a hermit. You begin singing "Praise the Lord." I witnessed this even in healthy people during the AIDS era. The words of Dido Sotiriou[9] now came to mind, "Fear is

---

9   Dido Sotiriou (1909-2004), a Greek writer and journalist, author of the novel

more powerful than death. One does not fear death, one is frightened of fear. Fear is now in command. It tramples upon humanity. It starts from the surface and reaches to the heart."

I existed to eat, take pills and become a monster. It was not the life I had imagined and I could not think of a reason to try to perpetuate it. If I had the right to choose, I would have preferred to die the very next day. Yet my mother insisted that all would change soon since science today performs miracles. "They will find a cure, it is only a matter of time."

We were a family on the edge, but united. We looked after each other carefully as if afraid that without taking notice we would lose one another. "It is all my fault," I would say to myself. "Such an idiot, stupid, worthless and laughable. We were the most envied family and now we have fallen apart. At least I will try not to die, that would bring them to their end too." This slowly became my obsession, not to die. They seemed content to have me around even as a zombie. My hospital and newspaper visits were the only traces of social life that I had left.

My years of taking Norvir, I cannot recall how many, two or three, ended in 1999 with my second bout of an acute intestinal infection. Every time I was hospitalized, day and night my mother would not leave my side. When my brother Stathis came to visit he would stay for hours and we would laugh at all the silly things he would say. Nothing could change our usual habits. My brother would leave, and we would then enjoy the serenity, in silence. After all, it was a miracle that we were still together. My father was unable to come to the hospital and got news of me by telephone.

When at home again we learned that Norvir was now available in syrup-form for easier consumption. This turned out to be unacceptable. I took the liquid which tasted like gasoline. I was unable to drink one drop. I told my doctor this and he replied it was either the syrup or taking shots. The pills were no longer available! My mother tasted it too, to help me decide. We understood it was for my own good but it was impossible for me to swallow the syrup a second time and the shots were out of the question. This became my first revolutionary step. I had heard of a better cocktail with Crixivan (another member of the protease inhibitor family) as the main component and two other pills which I do not remember the names, only that they did not require refrigeration.

I was comforted by this change. "Why had I not taken Crixivan from the start? I would have avoided the lipodystrophy of the Norvir," I thought then, trying to find a way to participate more actively in the decisions made for me. Slowly I regained my figure, becoming visually acceptable, and started visiting a health and beauty center in Athens. I became confident and even began a new relationship the following year. That was an important test for me because during the Norvir years I had forgotten my femininity. I felt nothing, not female or male, possibly neutral, indifferent, soul-less. It sounds unbelievable but I even moved in with my new boyfriend in the beginning of 2000. He was

Farewell to Anatolia (1962)

incredibly easy, intrepid, strong, healthy and feared nothing. He was also four years younger than me. He knew my story and either admired or pitied me. My mother viewed my new situation with an obvious satisfaction. It was a sign of my recovery. The doctors also seemed to be satisfied with their deeds.

I lived with Mario Tsirgiotis for one year, during which my hair started falling out; we would find them in every corner of the house, although fortunately I was not left bald. I awoke one morning in 2001, it was Christmas again, and I was speaking incoherently, banging and tossing my blankets and clothes in a state of frenzy. No one was prepared for this and Mario called the ambulance. I woke up two days later in the emergency ward of the General Hospital. It was my first case of meningitis, attributed to a virus related to the 'HIV' infection. It passed relatively fast, in a month or so, despite its noisy and vigorous manifestation. My condition remained precarious, so I felt the need to return home. Actually my mother took over the move, because my health became seriously unstable. A new period of neurological problems had arisen with the notorious Crixivan.

I soon discovered that I could not manage to articulate what I wanted to say and, another surprise to me, while trying to do so I would forget what it was about. At the end I could not even open the front door to my house because the key trembled uncontrollably in my hand. Something else also occurred, unrelated to the trembling. The frying pan fell from my hand into the sink just before I began frying, as if something inside was giving the wrong commands. I could not manage even to sign my name at the bank no matter how hard I tried. It was impossible to steer my hand correctly; "Let me sign for you," a kind teller had told sympathetically. I could not do simple errands.

I collapsed one day in the street and was picked up by the corner restaurant owner. He took me inside and waited for me to regain consciousness. "You fainted," he said, but I saw he was much too frightened for it to be a simple faint. I learned later, after repeated incidents, that I was now suffering from small epileptic seizures. One more nightmare, short-lived, as if being struck by lightning. You are traumatizing others, my mother said. Naturally I remembered nothing afterwards and could not know when I would be traumatizing people. It was a constant fear, even at home. "The epileptic seizures will not necessarily become permanent," explained the neurologist, "they are possibly caused only under certain conditions." I was given another combination of pills. My seizures ceased but something new appeared. I had double vision. I also told this to the neurologist who had become my second doctor, besides the AIDS colleagues. "Ah, you have double vision," he explained and changed my neurological treatment which always accompanied AIDS medication.

"Be patient, my dear. The doctors are doing their best," my mother was saying again. Over time the double vision became blurred. My condition peaked Christmas of 2002 when I was transported in the usual way to the hospital in a coma. Once again I had startled everyone in the middle of the night. "Mom, do you regret giving birth to me?" I asked her upon awaking and found her next to me. "Never, you have given me the greatest joy and now you're fighting such a battle alone, what can I do for you?"

She could do nothing. Once more they could not detect which microbe had infected me for 3 to 4 weeks. I felt I would not be waiting much longer, I had already "left" and was happy. I saw myself looking back at various stages of my life as if watching a film. I was bright, smiling, had a good life up until now. I opened my eyes and saw my mom at the distance of a breath. "It's over," is all I said, and saw her nodding the head. I wanted to say "thank you" but no one heard it. Dr. Kordosis recruited a special neurological professor from another hospital. He came dressed in a suit, it was the weekend. "Her condition is quite critical and the problem is that she is not communicating her symptoms to us," he had told my mother earlier. "We can promise nothing," the new neurologist said.

One day the doctors appeared wearing suspicious smiles. After repeated examinations they managed to track down the microbe, it was apparently TB, tuberculous meningitis. It was the worst that could happen to me but at least now they knew which antibiotic to give me. I began yet another "aggressive" treatment and when I recovered in the hospital I had no idea where I was, requesting one morning to have coffee and cookies on the veranda. I had completely lost it. I remember though how much I longed for it, a coffee and cookies on the veranda seeming like one of the greatest joys in life. My brother had come to the hospital and I did not recognize him. Various people would enter my room and I did not see them, I was later told. At some point towards the end of this hospitalization, I got out of bed and saw myself in the mirror. I was frightened by what I saw. I was no longer myself. I had turned grey, my face an ominous shadow, dull like a corpse. "You were 'being consumed' quite a bit every day, that's why TB is called phthisis (consumption)," explained my doctor.

I stayed at home, never going out, for a long time after that. Getting out of bed and going to the kitchen or bathroom was an exploit. My mother would help me shower. For many days she laid next to me telling stories so I would not despair. Little by little I started to recover. But I had to change my AIDS treatment since it was interferring with my TB treatment. When I was released from the hospital I had to take two, four and six pills daily – morning, afternoon and evening – instead of three, six and nine pills daily of the main AIDS medication for three months. I continued this until September of 2003 when I collapsed again. "How many pills per day are you taking?" I was asked. "Two, four, six," I answered. "That is wrong, we said to start again three, six and nine after three months. You are disturbing your treatment and we cannot be held responsible for the results," my doctor concluded truly angered. "Her problem is her lack of discipline," he explained to my mother, putting her in charge of maintaining the proper pill administration.

I recovered to a sustainable state after changing my pills to three, six and nine. I ventured outside my home and was pleased at getting around with relevant ease, so I restarted the visits to the beauty institute for face/ body treatment, electro therapies and more. The following year, in the beginning of 2004, I decided to start Latin dance lessons – to celebrate a little. With a pounding heart I would give it my all for about one hour at the school party. I would return home with no delay to enjoy my personal triumph a little bit longer. I had fooled everyone. At the dance school they had no idea about me, I was just another beginner, awkward but determined. There were even worse students than me.

I began appearing for work at the newspaper again. Everyone greeted me as if I had been resurrected, I was faking being OK and would not stay for long. It was Nikos Bakounakis who would say to me now: "I have a good topic for you, do you think you can have it done by Monday?" It was like oxygen, I would then go home and do my best to live up to his expectations.

However, though I had not really cried so much as long as I was waiting to die, now that there was a serious possibility that I would remain deficient like that – "almost well" - for the rest of my life, I was endlessly crying at home.

I managed to secure a place of my own, in the apartment above that of my parents, and there I could cry and cry undisturbed. Watching small injustices on the news, I would feel personally affected. When they started showing the tortures in Iraq, I was inconsolable. Undetectable to others, confusion began taking over my brain and I started losing parts of my memory. I felt insecure about everything and I was getting dizzy often. I would hide this at home by sitting in a chair motionless until I would recover. I had done the same at dance school several times, but now I could not even go there.

The horizon would disappear before me. Even walking down the street was dangerous. It was unbelievable. In order to cross Panepistimiou Street,[10] I asked for the arm of a lady next to me. To walk down the stairs at Syntagma Square was like going on the edge of a cliff. I stood in awe of any staircase, whether I needed to go up or down. It would sway in front of me, disappearing into a deep abyss. I got brain disease after the meningitis, my doctor explained to me, the virus had now reached the brain. My condition had worsened to the point that they feared I had got brain cancer.

"You did not come to my office so I could inform you," complained Dr. Kordosis to my mother. "I did not come because I know what you want to tell me, you have said it before. I cannot believe she has brain cancer, I DO NOT WANT to believe it." A consultation then took place at the doctor's office in the hospital which included me. They suggested a biopsy of my brain, assuming we would accept this solution. I had given up any defences but my mother reacted intensely. What if they hit a wrong nerve, then what? It was a fairly new procedure in our country. There was not much experience with the procedure making it quite risky. Once more I was taken aback with her effort to keep me alive in my pathetic state.

Thus we decided to go to London for a second opinion. Dr. Kordosis agreed to complete the paperwork necessary for my insurance to cover the expenses. He recommended the best neurological hospital, informing the doctors there that I would be coming, giving us some hope of salvation.

---

10 Panepistimiou Street: major street in central Athens

My 2004 visit to London was the beginning of yet another rebirth for me, despite the fact that it could be my last visit anywhere. I gathered up all traces of courage I had left and gave in completely to my brother's guidance for three intense days of meeting with the specialists at St. George's Hospital in London. Our fame had arrived before us. The first thing I was asked by the doctors there was, "Where is your mother?" We laughed. "Her English is not very good, she did not come," I said and we were able to regroup. My brother and another Greek doctor, G. P. would be the interpreters, since I could remember hardly anything. Dr. P. had been part of the Dr. K. team and was finishing another degree in London.

Using my medical records and the information given now, the director of the neurological clinic, Dr. R.H., and the professor of pathology-infections, G.E.G., catalogued my medical past in a very thorough British manner. For example, about the memory loss, they wrote, "Slowly she has realized that her amnesia has advanced considerably the last two years. She cannot recall faces and names, telephone numbers and birthdays. Her results on the IQ test were good but exhibits a certain weakness recalling what she witnessed five minutes ago. She remembered only two of the ten pictures we presented to her earlier. Even though she is employed at one of the biggest newspapers in Athens where she is a book critic, she is no longer confident about her work. The newspaper office has been transferred to a new building six months ago and she still cannot remember the new address and telephone number, according to her brother. Along with the memory loss, she admits to a certain amount of stress and symptoms of agoraphobia, low disposition, without panic attacks. She avoids social encounters yet still continues with Latin dance lessons. When she has to write a book review she works for four to five hours but needs one to two days to recover from the exhaustion. She exhibits trembling in her hands and some difficulties in mobility." They filled in the rest of the current image. "She talks clearly, speaks proper English, appears slightly stressed and breathes heavily with each pause." I remember being seated for one to two hours in a chair facing the English doctor. I wouldn't say much, but gave my best efforts.

In my medical records they first recorded signs of brain damage in 2002 and reported it was atrophying and worsening up to 2004. What had induced this catastrophe? The doctors noted that they had examined the possibility of toxic poisoning from the antiretroviral therapy. For some reasons incomprehensible to me, such as the lack of swelling in the brain which would suggest such an outcome, they assumed that poisoning had not occurred and, since they found no cyst or infection, they concluded that it was probably a classic case of HIV brain disease.

I repeated the same exams thatI had already done at least 15 times, since the equipment was more up to date. They decided to rule out the definitely risky brain biopsy and suggested the new drug Stocrin, which they said would deter the advancement of the virus in the brain. "We are not magicians that can make miracles happen. Your condition is irreversible, try to get strong by Christmas, if possible," I heard my diagnosis being catapulted at me again. It was November of 2004 and miraculously, when I stopped taking Crixivan and began the Stocrin, my nervous system started to recover. "It is the first time since you became ill that we are having a Christmas holiday like normal people," my brother commented joyously at the Christmas table. By February of 2005, I had reappeared at the dance school.

In reality, the drug Stocrin, which was less toxic than the previous medications (not a protease inhibitor, and not in the AZT category), allowed me to recover from their poisoning effect that the AIDS doctors had attributed to the 'HIV infection'. The only obvious side-effect I had was incredibly vivid action dreams, with strong images of terror, chases and death. They were so real that I would wake up startled and it would take some time for me to realize that it was only a dream.

This lasted for a few months, but at least I felt that I was slowly filling in my memory gaps. Scenes from the past were reappearing in my brain along with facts, information and names. It was surprising how many things I could recall from previously erased periods of time. Had I escaped danger then? I could not be sure, reassessing my new strength. I could drive again, exercise, dance and take long walks. Only my body had not come completely back to its shape. The lipodystrophy was still present in the same spots. Also my head often felt heavy and resting was difficult. Disappointment for me once more.

That Christmas my father died unexpectedly. Although he had a heart condition, it was cancer that took him within one month of being diagnosed. We had never revealed my condition to him. Could he have known? This misfortune became a catalyst for my family. My brother suggested something seemingly odd. "How about creating a web page so you can reach out to others?" During the two days following the funeral we took our first steps. We found the ideal contact – a colleague of my brother, named Manos Vassilakis – and made an agreement. By New Year's Eve, www.hivwave.gr was started.

What happened afterwards seems incredible, as if my father were pulling strings from heaven.

Chapter 4

Apocalypse: How I was saved

1. First came the hope

My presence on the Internet as an HIV-positive journalist who asked impertinent questions brought rapid results, mostly after I discovered the website www.PeaceandLove.ca and received an email from its 45-years-old Canadian webmaster, Gilles Saint-Pierre. A big change happened in my life with his arrival in Athens on April 23, 2006. I didn't expect him to save me at all, but was living the new reality as a dream. What my new friend had already written to me was exceptional; one of his quotes for instance:

> I believe the more love there is in the world, the less violence. And I'm not just talking here about love of humankind. That's a wonderful, very important kind of "altruistic" love, but it can only go so far because it's not passionate (and who the hell wants to go to bed with all of humankind anyway?). Violence is passionate. It can only be defeated by an equally passionate, powerful force like romantic erotic love. [11]

He had studied biology at the university and had systematically dealt with the AIDS hypothesis. He found me charming in the pictures and in the exchange of mails, and was probably thinking of comforting me when he wrote in another mail that he would like to be the father of my child – I didn't take it seriously. He seemed to mean it from the start, though. "You have nothing bad", he was trying to convince me that HIV virus does not exist, "Either named HIV or something else, something infected me", I would answer. "Nothing infected you ever", he would say. "But I was sick for ten years", I would reply.

He would then try to explain that the stress related to the positive HIV test unconsciously caused the first 'AIDS disease', since I believed in it, and the pills I had agreed to take did the rest. That is, I had somehow caused all that catastrophe on my own. When he concluded like that, I felt anger simmering inside. "Other people around me have more stress and they don't become sick", I would insist.

It was a little bit difficult for me to believe what he was saying but, judging

---

[11] *Chemistry of Love* by Dr. Susan Block, CounterPunch, February 12 / 13, 2005

by the end result, I would say that Gilles played the role of the therapist I never had. The goal of therapy is to assist the patient to reconnect the broken pieces of the self. From Canada, Gilles provoked me with his questions, and his subsequent arrival in Greece then conquered me. I felt obliged to respond. What an experience! He extracted details from me. Together we made the connections, expanding the limits of our freedom. Soon we got married, became a real couple.

I wondered how he could love me, with the traces of ten years of hardship evident upon me and the side effects of the medicine still there, notwithstanding how well I had learned to deal with them. He had learned how to drift with me then, he would word everything obliquely: "I don't see anything strange, maybe you are missing a little fat here..." How sweet! Little by little I would become more open, I loved his attention, he would not stop taking care if he thought I was still suffering.

I began to see myself through Gilles' eyes. I didn't feel exactly like a dream spouse, although hoping for better with time. Whatever task I would start, my strength would quickly abandon me, even eating became a chore. "Not this again," my mother would say while cooking the best food, always there for us. The problem was not so much the food but my back. It could not support me for long when I sat at the table. I wanted either to be moving or lying down, like I was before. Mostly I didn't sleep well during the night, it was impossible to find any comfortable position for my legs, because they were aching at the joints. I was waiting for the dawn to jump out of bed. Perhaps I only seemed lazy the rest of the day.

It was always possible that my condition might worsen at any time. The different AIDS medications seemed to affect a different part of the body every time. As soon as I would change treatments, my symptoms from the previous one would disappear and shortly thereafter new symptoms would appear somewhere else in my body. In between there would be a period of rest from the hostilities. Each therapy needed some time to manifest its negative self. Perhaps I was in one of those in-between periods. I didn't want even to think of it, since Gilles wouldn't complain. Every now and then, though, he would say: "Why don't you read any of the books I brought? " I had tried to, by all means. He had brought an entire suitcase of books filled with evidence of the truth and I did not know where to begin and what conclusion to draw.

2. Then came the questions

I pulled out a book called *Inventing the AIDS Virus,* written by Peter Duesberg, with a prologue from the Nobel Prize winner Kary Mullis, from a special shelf on Gilles' bookcase. It was here that I read the following:[12]

Despite Gallo's repeated booms and busts, virus hunting was the

---

12 Duesberg, Inventing the AIDS virus, Regnery Publishing 1966 pp. 125-6.

fashion, and he doggedly pursued retroviruses for the next few years. In 1980 he finally reported having found the first known human retrovirus. The virus was isolated from human leukemia cells grown for a long time in the lab, with no immune system to interfere or suppress the virus. Gallo's team even had to shock the cells repeatedly with potent chemicals to coax the soundly sleeping virus out of latency. No such virus could be found in a second batch of leukemic cells, but Gallo remained unfazed, giving the new virus a name with strong propaganda value – Human T-cell Leukemia Virus, or HTLV …

HTLV researchers can change other rules, too. Having first assumed the virus is spread between adults, scientists calculated a "latent period" of five years between infection and development of leukemia. Soon they adjusted that figure to ten years, then thirty, as they found increasing numbers of healthy carriers of HTLV. Once they decided the virus is transmitted sexually, though leukemia strikes roughly at age sixty, they subtracted twenty from sixty to generate a forty year-latent period. Then upon realizing that the virus is actually transmitted from mother to child around birth, the latent period grew to an official forty to fifty-five years.

My skin crawled when I thought of what all this could mean, I did not dare to believe it could be so false because my experience was quite real. However, I knew much about Dr. Duesberg who had been nominated for the Nobel Prize for his ground-breaking work on fighting cancer and had been honored repeatedly for his research at the University of California at Berkeley . He was shunned and slandered when he started expressing his objections to the HIV/AIDS hypothesis in 1987, like a Galileo of the 20th century.

He was among the ones who had shown interest in me when I started communicating with the universe of "dissidents" overseas. Yes, the renowned Dr. Peter Duesberg had put one more little stone in my liberation path, with two simple questions. The first was sent to me by email, on December 15th 2006: "Maria, do you take anti-HIV drugs?" And then I replied properly:

Dr Duesberg, I'm thrilled to have a message from you! Anti-HIV drugs, I've taken almost all of them. 1985: first diagnosed HIV-positive, I told no one, took no medication. 1995: second time diagnosed HIV-positive after a pneumonia, sent to the proper hospital, took Septra and AZT, ended with anemia and cytomegalovirus. 1996: Norvir and two others, ended with viral meningitis and tuberculosis meningitis. 2000: Crixivan and two others, ended with short epileptic crisis and encephalopathy. 2004: Stocrin, almost reborn however easily tired, and started a new life with the website www.hivwave.gr and writing two books at once. I'm newly married with non-HIV-positive Gilles St-Pierre, webmaster of www.peaceandlove.ca, who believes that I should stop the medications. My doctors, together with my mother and brother, beg me to continue or else it will be a clearly suicidal action. I think it is an impasse. You made me happy with your communication, The best to you too.

He replied:
> Dear Maria, Thanks for your response. Now I have a second question: What AIDS-defining illnesses are you currently suffering from? Based on the pictures on your website you look very healthy to me. Cordially, Peter D.

Was he possibly implying that I could get rid of the pills? I didn't know how to answer, I needed time to assimilate such a thing, to persuade my family, but I could not keep such a scientist waiting for me to decide. Besides, since Gilles was not successful in that, nobody would be. So I reluctantly stopped that exchange.

In the aftermath, I would peruse some of the books Gilles had brought and return them, again disappointed. Since I had lived the disease, how could those authors claim that it does not exist? My beloved had also brought a film called *"The Other Side of AIDS,"* a 2004 documentary containing numerous testimonies from HIV positives, and asked the obvious of me, that we watch it together. However, after starting the video, I would leave by the middle, "I know all this, I've been through it, I don't need to see it again".

In June we went to Canada on our honeymoon. It was there that Gilles played the documentary for his sister and his brother-in-law, and called me into the room to join them. I did not utter a word as I watched it till the end. I saw HIV-positive people who had taken the AIDS drugs and were like me now, though others who did not take them had stayed healthy. And I saw Kary Mullis saying:

> I mean it was a bizarre thing that happened. It really was. It didn't really have any precedence in terms of medicine before that. Unless perhaps you could think of the possession by devil stuff, right? You see, once you're possessed by the devil, anything that happens to you or anything you do is -- has got to do with that, right? You don't suddenly notice that one new organism is causing every problem.

I would smile contentedly, but that was not enough. Was it possible for me now to go back to step one? Feelings of euphoria and rage would intermix while I was writing my second book in Canada, *The game of love in the time of AIDS*, to define the new unexpected state of well-being. I would end with the conclusion that "I cannot stop the therapy I have taken for the past ten years, it could be risky to bring another shock to my organism". Yet, deep inside, I hoped to change my mind.

Back in Athens, I read a book by the protagonist of the documentary, Christine Maggiore, titled *What if Everything You Knew About AIDS Was Wrong?*[13] I found in there the definition of what had happened to me, after all:

---

13 Christine Maggiore, What if Everything You Knew About AIDS Was Wrong? 1996,

Can you imagine receiving a fatal diagnosis without being told the diagnosis is based on an unproven idea and an uncertain test? Being instructed to take powerful, experimental drugs without being told these drugs compromise health, destroy functions necessary to sustain life, and were approved for use without adequate testing? Being informed that you have, or should expect, deadly illnesses without being told that these same illnesses are not considered fatal when they occur in "normal" people?

Now the euphoria together with anger would set in for good. And, even worse, I didn't know who to blame for that, how to explain what had happened. Maggiore had already described in 1996 the mistake of my life - soon after Duesberg's book, and I had missed those important news items, although I was supposedly in a centre of the information world (a journalist in the book section of the largest newspaper in Greece)? "She discovered she was 'HIV positive' in 1992 but reacted quicker than you have, because she lived in Los Angeles, a breath away from many of the dissidents in the US", Gilles tried to comfort me.

All these years I imagined that suspicious scientists had constructed something and I thought it was kept a secret and would be so forever, since no one in the world press seemed to be capable of uncovering it. Gilles would enlighten me again: They did not keep their creation a secret but rather advertised it, "Everyone get tested." Actually, the only thing that has spread since 1984 seemed to be the HIV-antibody test, together with the belief that there is a lethal virus called HIV that is transmitted sexually, etc. And the myth was reinforced with appalling reports of AIDS in Africa and even today there are distracting ideas being fostered that there are government agents behind the creation of a virus to annihilate black Americans and to obliterate the homosexuals of the Western world. Anyway, a new disease did not appear on the horizon, just new names. And latest news, latest news, latest news.

I thought that they certainly could have created the test to condemn those the Western world considered high risk and their intimate partners, for no one knows what it detects and how it was manufactured. "It detects simple antibodies, anyone can have positive results," protested Gilles. "So, again, how was he negative and I positive?" At this point we could argue forever. In the end the conclusion for me was the same: maybe it was time to quit the medication I had been taking for so many years?

I started discussing the issue at home but it was not an easy task to convince my family. I did not have the right to hurt them again. They had seen for years the best doctors in Athens fighting for me, had spent endless nights in the hospital, having practically lost all hope and now finally seeing me married to a wonderful man. I was happy and smiling again. Why push it? I did not feel certain either. Just the thought of returning to the emergency ward of the hospital only to be probed again to find what had infected me this time caused me much despair. I wanted my peace of mind and my present happiness even with the prospect of dying the next day – so to speak.

Besides, Gilles had still to answer the same persistent question, if he wanted me to be persuaded. How is it that, in 1995, I was found in the last stages of AIDS? Why did I have a prolonged fever that would not fall? He had said from the start that it was due to stress, but I could still not understand how stress can cause pneumonia.

My significant other found a short and clear answer this time, within many of the emails we were receiving from all over the world. Michael Geiger, member of the organization HEAL (Health, Education, AIDS, Liaison), gave indirectly the answer to that particular question:.

> Do a Google search for "stress" and "thymus gland." You will find that the thymus is where your CD4 T-cells are born, you will find it is the center of your immune system and you will find that stress causes it to shut down in less than 24 hours. Stress shuts down the immune system. Be it chemical stresses, emotional stresses, physical stresses including the stress of lack of nutrition or toxic drinking water, or the extreme and acute fear and panic type of stress of an HIV or AIDS diagnosis. Stress shuts down the thymus. Stress causes AIDS. In every case of AIDS you will find obvious and non-obvious high stressors. Some are even subconscious. Stress=AIDS, not food, acidic or otherwise. Period. And that is my own take on AIDS, though you are welcome to believe as you will.

"That's it! The emotional, subconscious stress could not be detected in any of the exams made in the Medical Center", Gilles said. "That is why they had received negative results in all their tests, before the 'HIV' one". We also heard Dr. Val Turner from the Perth Group in Australia in a short video explaining that the emotion accompanied with the news of a death sentence exhausts the immune system alarmingly fast.

In retrospect, I would say now it was a hidden stress that placed me on the sickly AIDS path, the exhausting psychological stress of being HIV positive – though I had never admitted it, not even to myself. I would say "Don't let it defeat you", but could not stop the unconscious impact of hopelessness. "When you stop hoping, you start dying", Gilles said. So, that explains my deteriorating health in the years before I started on the useless but toxic 'AIDS' medication.

Medical experts should know that, if there was really a free flow of information. "Numerous experiments, that had been conducted for some decades now, had shown that severe and chronic psychological stress can cause symptoms very similar to the ones we meet today with AIDS – notably the fall in CD4 numbers and the occurrence of illnesses such as pneumonia, tuberculosis, emaciation, dementia", as I finally found in the book by Dr Etienne de Harven & Jean-Claude Roussez "*Les 10 plus gros mensonges sur Le Sida*" (2005). The suspicion and fear that you may have been "infected", since you believe in the HIV=AIDS hypothesis, is enough to finish you off even if you did not do the test.

I was feeling frustrated by Gilles' discoveries. For the first time in this journey, I shuddered to think.

3. Just a decision taken

It was the beginning of 2007, on one of our last visits to the private office of Dr. T.K. with my sweetheart, that we had inquired if we could have children. I had asked the same question in the past when I was with Mario and the answer had been "Yes," perhaps because he then hoped for a better outcome from my therapy. We never had a chance, I was afflicted with meningitis soon after. I had now overcome the hurdles, I proved resilient and felt a new confidence when we went to the doctor. Although Gilles had ruled out child birth for me while still on drugs, I wanted to know the doctor's opinion.

"The child will be fine" he responded, "however, without a mother". Excuse me? Without a mother? Up until now we knew the opposite, with the new medication I would live happily. This doctor was always concise and now he was actually giving me the greatest gift – he confirmed what non-doctors were telling me about the risks of the medication. But did he have to say it so clear? He had not been so blunt since 1995.

On the side walk of Vasilissis Sofias avenue, my sweetheart took me with his two hands, lifted me like a small child and kissed me lovingly. I felt as if escaping from a sinking ship. We crossed the avenue to Mavili Square and sat in front of the fountain which began fluttering with a soft frrrr. Up until then it had been silent and as soon as we appeared its jets suddenly began to dance. The world around us changed as if our meeting with the doctor had never taken place. We watched the children staring in bewilderment at the fountain, the mothers who kept an eye on them, the old ladies sipping on their coffee in the background and the strolling couples, with a husband proud to accompany his pregnant wife. From where had they all sprouted? Had we been blind until now? We exchanged glances and pondered when we would join the club.

In the taxi on our way home the thought entered my mind again as to how we were going to convince my mother to take yet another journey into the unknown. "Maria, you'd rather stop taking AIDS medication. I will send you each week some of my publications in which you will see why I recommend this," I remembered a series of recent e-mails from my latest ally, in Chicago, Dr. Andrew Maniotis. I would eagerly read through his e-mails waiting for the next one as if I was under a spell, unable to do anything else. This new ally was a second generation Greek-American from Mani[14] in the Peloponnese, Director of the Laboratory for Cell and Developmental Biology of Cancer at the University of Illinois, Chicago, a teacher in one of the largest medical schools in the USA and he was clearly on my side.

---

14 Mani, the middle peninsula of the Peloponnese, famed for the independent nature of its inhabitants, for the tower houses and fortified family dwellings from the period of the Ottoman occupation of Greece.

He had even given me his telephone numbers in Chicago. Perhaps now I could make up for my pointless approach to Dr. Duesberg. I chose the appropriate time, one that would be morning on the other side of the Atlantic, picked up the phone mechanically and dialed Maniotis' office number. I was certain it was he who answered the phone. "Hello I am Maria Papagiannidou from Athens, from Greece...." He was happy to speak with me and asked if I could spend some time on the phone discussing things with him. He was informative as usual, his facts being however purely scientific. "My mother will never agree," I revealed the severe obstacle at the end. "Do not tell your mother," was his response in its familiar tone. Yet it echoed like an alarm, "You are in danger!"

Nothing could hold me now, I went directly to my mother. I related to her, not only my telephone conversation with Dr. Maniotis, but also the recent events with our doctor. "Inadmissible," she said. I replied: "It means I quit the AIDS medication". Silence. I took the two pill bottles and discarded them in the trash. "Don't throw them away, you may change your mind," my mother shouted, always having foresight. "No way," I replied curtly. Curiously there were no more reactions, just surprise, the bottles were now history. I would never go again to fill my prescriptions. We needed the confirmation from a qualified medical scientist, we had it now. That was more than a gift from Dr. Maniotis. "You know that I will stand by you, whatever decision you may take", Mom soon said. Gilles had nothing else to add, but enjoyed watching our reactions. I was touched.

My glorious bilingual web page had won me international acceptance thanks to his interventions from Canada and Athens, and he waited for me patiently, regardless how strange my behavior could be. Even now, in making my decision, he showed understanding of what was going on inside of me, it was difficult to throw out the medication. I knew they cost the Greek nation so much. I had once been informed that each AIDS patient costs the government 1,000,000 drachmas (2,941 euro) per month, that is 35,294 euros per year. Such an ineffectual sacrifice was being made by the nation for us. Rather the Greek taxpayers were being sacrificed.

Naturally my sweetheart could not know that for so many years I had yearned anxiously for the pills and made sure I was supplied in time because sometimes they "ran out" in the storage room of the hospital as patients would come from out of town and stock up. Supplies were limited. Then I would lose it. Where is my medication? If you put a dent in my program I will go back to the hospital. Now where will I go? Go to Syngrou[15]. Who will I ask for there? I would then rush there with my car to get there before they closed their storage room. Would they have extra for me? Whenever I succeeded, a feeling of relief would overcome me. So many successive mistakes? I would tell all this to Gilles now. As I unveiled what had occurred each time, I felt myself getting free of it. I slowly began regaining confidence in myself.

---

15 Syngrou, a major hospital of Athens

Surprisingly, things seemed to happen on their own from that point on. I stopped the pills on St. George's Day and that evening we were to go to our best man's house, George Papaioannou, Villi's husband, for a party. No one there knew of that day's decision. Towards the end of the evening George pulled me up to dance disco, I thought of declining but could not. With each turn I thought I would fall. Most likely because that is what I thought, not because it would actually happen. I never fell, and wrote about the evening to Dr. Maniotis, who replied:

> "The leg weakness is a symptom reported by many many people on the meds as being the first indication of peripheral neuropathy due to the drugs. The fact that you can still walk is somewhat of a miracle – but if you can dance the night away, I'm sure you are going to be fine. In fact, disco dancing late into the night after a few glasses of wine to solubilize the fat in your body would be just what the doctor ordered as a form of detox, and mental balance. Dance into a sweat as much as you can, in addition to doing all the other things. I am so glad you are doing so well-but then again, after I heard about the details, I had no doubts that you are going to be fine."

So there is the difficult part of the story, dancing disco every night! He probably meant going to a gym, but that had already been in my weekly program for years. I laughed every time I would read a new message from the honourable Dr. Maniotis

Nothing noteworthy happened the following day, only a pleasurable void inside me, in my stomach and my head. I felt lighter. I understood suddenly how tense I had been for so long. Perhaps I would not be able to do a good job at work? Only time would tell. I had only to be careful to conceal my new situation, because there existed a danger of instigating panic amongst those close to me. Once again the same AIDS scenario appeared, having to watch out whom I spoke to or not. I told a couple of friends on the telephone and they froze, "Why did you do that?!! With the new pills you were fine..." Everyone knows that the war against AIDS has consumed more money and human effort than a trip to the moon. I would be able to cope better by myself? "I am worried about you..." I was told by a few friends. I remembered something I had heard in the documentary *AIDS: Fact or Fiction?* "Those people who are HIV positive are victims of society who kill them by their prejudice before the drugs with the particular side-effects." I had to cut out some people along with the drugs for a little bit longer.

Certainly there was no time for explanation to everyone as we now wished to speed up the process as much as possible. I was now impatient, back to myself. The next day I only thought not to take my scooter to work, for to stop such a harsh treatment is no small feat. I went hesitantly to work thinking I had a label on my forehead saying "I quit medication." No one seemed to notice. The next day I drove my scooter again, carefully. I went, came back, and everything was fine. Soon I would be able to reveal it to Andy – that is how he,

Dr. Maniotis, had signed his last mail to me.

I had waited some time before sending him the news ten days later. Given the opportunity, I now asked if I could have children since I was no longer taking drugs. The answer I received on the 17th of May was, in my words, "Go for it!" In his words, it was the following:

> Dear Maria,
>
> I don't see why not have a baby. But I'd wait until you feel confident that all those drugs are out of your system. You wouldn't want to expose your beautiful son or daughter to them! They have to grow up to be the new Greek Prime minister, the next Maria Callas, or at least Greece's future Olympic hopeful (or perhaps they will be a hated scientist some day). Just make sure they don't become doctors!
>
> The drugs you were taking all have warnings that pregnancy while taking the drugs is contraindicated (you shouldn't do it). But in time, all that poison will be eliminated from your fat and other toxin storage areas (bones, nervous system, and especially your hair follicles and hair). I do have some knowledge about what is called "clearance" of toxins from the body. You can hasten (speed up) the process of detoxification by doing steam-baths or jacuzzi regimens, and there are all kinds of detoxifying regimens you can try that do work to eliminate all toxins from the body. In fact, if I were you, I'd do this even if you didn't want to have a baby, for your own health.
>
> I am 49 and have had 3 beautiful children, and two of them are nearly on their own. Please let me give you some advice (and also to Gilles). Before you decide to have a child, I would strongly suggest that you guys enjoy some time together as a couple who are in effect survivors of a Nazi death camp – the AIDS death camp. Give yourselves some time to fall in love and interact as non-stigmatized, non-diseased, normal people again, as it probably was when you guys met.
>
> When the press or when anyone finds out that you are pregnant, you could be besieged by something that is worse than a Nazi occupation (like the US in Iraq). Read Christine's story about how she was breast-feeding Charlie, and Eliza Jane (when she was alive) and the shit she had to endure from the AIDS spinners in the press, and elsewhere. It was disgusting! A mother can't raise her own child the way she wants if she in any way shape or form has any connection to "HIV."
>
> I suggest you give yourself some time to prepare for this possibility, or, just prepare for the ordeal that parenting itself will bring. Parenting is a great deal of fun, and all parents cannot help becoming better human beings because of their children. Allowing some time before pregnancy will as I say also be good for your eventual child (may she be as pretty as you are or as strong-looking as Gilles), and it will give you some much needed time to return to living "NORMAL" again.

But these are just words and advice from an "old" young man.
Love,
  Andreas (Andy Maniotis)

It was now the beginning of June and one month had passed with no medication. I witnessed it everyday in the mirror: my face was more vibrant. Others noticed it too, but they could not imagine the reason. "You look beautiful, what are you doing?" asked Vili, the mother of my godson who had recently seen me at her house party. I was the possessor of an amazing secret and apparently it showed.

I then revealed to her all the details, as I used to do in the past, in difficult situations and in our student years. She stared at me in suspense as if the news seemed unbelievable, as it did even to me. I continued to explain to her that I simply needed to eat ten oranges a day and take hot baths or sauna to expel the toxins from my body – these were my first instructions. The ten oranges were soon switched to a few glasses of fresh squeezed juice. Most importantly, my detoxification ritual gave me time to dream again and the happiness was showing in my eyes. My friend was stunned but kept skeptical for a while.

Gilles and I contemplated how to prepare the Athenian society for this stunning news. I had already been unexpectedly given one of the "Excellence" awards in the ceremony "Women of the Year 2006" that is organized every year by the magazine *Life and Style*. Of course I did not then know that my glorious emancipation was to follow, yet somewhere inside me I felt it approaching and in some ways I exuded it. The director of the magazine, Christos Zabounis, happened to know of me professionally from my work at the *To Vima* newspaper and entrusted the journalist Aggeliki Papadopoulou to interview me for the magazine, to talk about my life.

He and his readers were inspired by my brief account, and the same occurred at the Athens Arena where I received my award in a packed hall in front of a mixed crowd who gave me a standing ovation. Some were quite displeased by this response. "You do not know what you are doing, you are not a doctor to judge this woman's actions," were just some of the many harassing words that Christos received. "Ne t'inquiete pas," he said to relieve me in front of Gilles, at another one of our meetings. He told to us some of the laughable occurrences that followed the ceremony, and said "Don't worry. I do not give any importance to such things."

We presented Gary Null's documentary "*AIDS Inc.*" at the movie theatre "Microkosmos" in Athens in May 2007. However it was organized rapidly and only had a small turnout. Mostly it was just my good friends who attended, and they left the movie theater a bit confused.

We reviewed the four critical 'AIDS' documentaries that we had obtained from the US and Europe, in order to select the one that would be most convincing. We then organized a 15-day film presentation in Athens and other interested cities. We chose "*The Other Side of AIDS*" by Robin Scovill, the one I did not want to view originally, with Christine Maggiore as the main narrator. It had now become my favourite – an excellent film that won an award in the

Los Angeles International Film Festival. Without giving it a second thought, we sent the producers 2,000 US dollars for the copyright. Once we factored in the Greek subtitles for the film and its promotion, we had spent all of our vacation budget. Still, our life was then full of special moments.

We had a warm reception from the owners of the two cinemas in Athens, Andrea Sotirakopoulos at the "Microkosmos" and Leonida Papageorgiou at "Trianon", despite them starting to receive the familiar harassment, "What you are about to do is pure madness." We arranged the posters and the invitations in record time with the help of the enterprising "Oxy" publisher Nikos Hatzopoulos. We scheduled the preview and invited the most distinguished journalists, television personalities, writers, friends and acquaintances. By the end of June we were ready. The opening would be free and the following days five euros. "Whatever is free is looked on as unworthy," I had dogmatically decided. I even planned to give all the proceeds to the owners to cover the costs of the presentation. I was that sure. But again, very few people came to the opening, besides our closest friends. The turnout was also meagre for two weeks afterwards. "We failed to convince them that this was not just another documentary about AIDS", was our conclusion - but how could we ever achieve the opposite? People had become tired of the many different approaches to the subject matter.

The documentary had a better reception in Patra, where an old friend, Spiros Boulis, the owner of the radio station Sport FM Patras, organized our welcome. There was not a plethora of people but I was impressed by their interest and their touching reactions. The composer Sotiris Sakellaropoulos did not meet us in Patras but he heard about us and called in Athens. He wanted to send me a musical composition he thought suited me.

Gilles and I returned refreshed. Any disappointments we took as useful lessons for the future. What mattered was achieving our main goal. It appeared closer and closer since we were winning allies.

Andy was always there for us. He had written to me shortly before we left for Patras in July:

> Dear Maria,
>
> How are you feeling? Still eating oranges (orange juice) everyday I hope? I think that you should be getting energy and a feeling of "health" back by now. Severe alcoholism detox takes about 10 days, Valium addiction clearance takes about 2 months, Prozac clearance from the body takes about 5-8 months, and there are no good studies I know of regarding the detox duration necessary to clear AIDS drugs, but the natural turnover of cells in the body can be on the order of 6 months. Have you bought a hot tub yet? It has been about 1 month since you stopped (you said the 2nd of May was your last dose).
>
> Please keep me informed (if you want) about your progress. You are not only very brave to trust your own logic (and that of Gilles), but you obviously are an extremely intelligent and loving person that through your own instincts knew that you weren't "doomed". Your "How One AIDS Case Can Change The World" piece, and the TV

interview I saw you in talking to that woman journalist paints a picture of a beautiful, intelligent, and energetic Greek woman who is committed to freeing her people from the lies of the US government. And I am committed to helping you deliver the next Greek Nobel Laureate in the form of a son or daughter.

Such kind hearted words from someone I had never met. He was certain that I could achieve this goal, it was obvious. Regardless, his words were reinvigorating. His message continued,

I constantly think about coming to Greece, and starting all over. I would love to teach, for example, at The University of Athens, or work at EMBL in Heraklion, Crete. Better yet, if I could get support from scientists world wide (both Greeks and non-Greeks), I have fantasies about starting a new institute in Athens called, "The Institute for Cancer and Human Immunity." It wouldn't be all wet-bench research, but would involve committees of dedicated individuals who study problems relating to human and environmental health. I need to gather about 200 people who can contribute 1,000,000 dollars or some fraction of that to get such an initiative started. I have been asking folks for several years now if they have a similar fantasy they would like to see materialize. We would need researchers and writers as well as scientists, and perhaps people who do a variety of different things. I do so want to help Greece and feel I owe her something of great value or beauty before I die.

Do you know how proud I was when Greece threw the Olympic games several years ago? What a pageant! What a victory for Greece that Olympics turned out to be! Yet when I went there the following summer, the Greeks I talked to were sort of critical of what the successful presentation of the Olympics really amounted to - in the eyes of the world. It was truly fantastic, from the perspective of a Greek American, like me, and I would like to see that same kind of enthusiasm and perfection in all Greek endeavours-in Greek science, medicine, law, politics, etc.

Please, if you know people in Greek academics, don't hesitate to forward them my desires and plan to be of help to Greece. This country I live in currently is a lost cause, and will never recover, or not for a very long time recover, from the current Nazi regime damage that has occurred.

Cheers,
And eat an extra orange for me today!
Fondly,
Andy

I was re-energized. I had a mission to complete. Our psychological state truly does affect our bodily health! Suddenly the thought of imminent death had disappeared. It was not even a topic for discussion. I recalled a part from the documentary *"The Other Side of AIDS,"* which describes that exact opposite flow of events which was my life up until recently.   Michael Ellner, the president of HEAL in New York, hypnotherapist and author of the essay *"The Healing Power of Story Telling"*, was answering the question "What is the impact of being HIV positive?"

> Bone pointing is a phenomenon where in aboriginal groups there's a belief that someone in the group has the power of life and death. And if a member of the group breaks a taboo, this person has the power to hex them and kill them by pointing a bone. Now, this bone has killed many, many believers. But later on, when the missionaries came and when the Europeans came and these people were conquered, they pointed their bones at the missionaries. They pointed their bones at the soldiers. It had no power. Because the power of the bone was in the belief. And what made it work is it wasn't only the individual's belief, it was the whole community, the whole group shared this belief. Well, what I noticed when I started going to the different AIDS organizations, like GMHC and the people with AIDS Coalition or Body Positive and other groups like that, was if somebody said, you know, "I think I'm gonna live", everybody in the group said, "You're in denial. You' re gonna die". And so it seemed to me that the reinforcement came from everywhere they turned. The doctors expected them to die. Their loved ones expected them to die. The people in like situations expected them to die.

You are in "denial." How many times have I heard this, ever since I began to have a voice! I was supposed to remain mute and depressed. The first time I felt that was when I wrote the book *"Maria K, How I Defeated AIDS"*, and their intentions became clearer. "She thinks she has defeated it but she lives in denial," some HIV believers asserted.   I was even sent this message in consecutive repetition through mail on my web page. Up until then I had never seen this expression and found it somewhat paranoiac for so many to agree on what was happening to me. Now I know: this is regarded as the right answer to those who raise their heads against the almighty lords of AIDS. Probably it is part of the ritual associated with the AIDS religion.

They would have no power over me any more. My blessing was the appearance of other wise men, much more powerful. The bone was now held by Dr. Maniotis from Chicago. What a difference! He showed me I would have a good life. I would only listen to him and let others continue their song and dance. I knew now I had a new direction, the only one I saw in front of me.

I had to be cautious, though, with my bodily reactions and not be fooled by my enthusiasm. I wrote to Andy the truth: I now wake up tired, sleepy all day long, as if carrying a load still inside me.

He replied:

> Dear Maria, Some folks sleep for months after an injury. Your cells

have been injured. Let them heal. It takes time – you'll feel much much better two months from now. As always, Love, Andy

No other significant difficulty appeared. However, Andy suggested finding a naturopath, to take care of any health problem that could occur in 'seronegative' people. What if that specialization does not exists in this country? I would find a homeopathic doctor instead.

In the meantime I had began walking frequently, following that other prescription from my doctor. Walking would strengthen my bones and stimulate the immune system. I was taking vitamins from four different bottles and added garlic to my diet, cinnamon and some days a glass of red wine. I even found the homeopathic doctor I was searching for. I was referred to him by a new friend, who visited my web page. She told me he was excellent, saying he had assisted her detoxification from AIDS treatments. I was not even the first in Greece.

"You can make a difference now Maria. Many are watching you", Lambros Papantoniou, the Greek correspondent in Washington, a new friend, wrote to me. I had no objection, having lived through the cataclysm, I was not going to keep quiet.

But although I could not admit it, I was beginning to lose my patience. When would I tell myself that I had overcome it? With eyes closed I would imagine the end of the detoxification. I would open them and be still impatient. In the end I found a solution, I began writing this book.

How did Ellner put it? There is therapeutic power in writing your own story. As long as I write, I am not drowsy, even working overtime. I will be O.K. by the time the book is completed. I will do it with ultimate care, so that it become the best possible. It will also need its corrections. By the end of it, I will be absolutely fine.

4. Farewell to the system

What would I do about my doctors? For years they had been my guardian angels. I had not been mistaken, they loved me and proved so each time I needed their attention. They had come on a Saturday to the hospital and always searched for a way to relieve me. I thought what a profession it is to be a doctor. You appear like the sun to people who have sunk in the dark. I remember how I waited every day to see them enter my room around two in the afternoon for their regular visit. For months it was the only time of day that had any worth to me. These were essentially the first doctors of my life, for until then I recall having only taken aspirin. They appeared as giants, the only ones capable of handing the difficult cases of people who were HIV positive. What heroes!

And now they have to close their eyes and ears, to block out knowledge of their possible service to a deception. It is unfathomable if it is really true. We never discussed the essence of it all once the revelations began. What to include and what to omit in our encounters? I knew the doctors were the last ones responsible for the moral lapse in science. I still believe this.

However, I read with sadness all that I previously wrote for my website, "the medical attendant is a best friend for the HIV positive patient, having helped AIDS patients in calm and in strenuous times. I am not only referring to the medical approach to the situation. I am speaking of lifelong relationships, a personal connection, an unwritten contract between the positive patient and their doctor. Without exaggeration I would say the people are earthly gods. They exist and do not exist. They are omnipresent without being present and when I need them they appear and do miracles."

Now I never wanted to see them again. Yet I would not criticize them, for as I had been deceived, they had also been deceived. However there was a crucial difference between us, they were the experts of the situation, providing me with the best information and I, if I wanted to survive, had to believe them.

I could forget them all to avoid another disaster, but the revelations were falling from the sky and I cited them one after the other on my web page. It was becoming all the more contradictory, confusing. One reader wrote "how can you consider your doctors gods if AIDS is a deception?" As if the oddness of the situation were not enough, I began receiving information from all over Greece about nasty behavior from some AIDS doctors. The most spectacular case was of a doctor in Thessaloniki (Dr. B. K.) who "was 'dismissed' because of infringements and illegalities," as an anonymous HIV positive patient wrote to me.

I was later told of the alleged major mistakes that had terminated his position. He was said to have prescribed medication from only one pharmaceutical company at the expense of competitors. If so, he had probably been well compensated by that company. My doctors were not like that. They selected the latest medication every time to save me. It was the most they could do for me as AIDS specialists. Their mistake was to specialize in AIDS. I judge people by their intentions and they had the best. I do not recall my doctors going away on cruises paid for by big pharmaceutical corporations.

It appears that they still do not comprehend what is now happening around us. The human mind resists, I understand, It needs some preparation time. But once it has been accomplished, one wants to shout it to the world: we conquered! We emerged from the dark into the light. Perhaps you do not see clearly at first glance, but eventually you request a re-examination of everything all together! Rebecca Culshaw, a professor at the University of Texas, is that kind of person. In March 2006, she published an article entitled "Why I quit HIV,"[16] giving an account of her own evolution.

> Over the past ten years, my attitude towards HIV and AIDS has undergone a dramatic shift. This shift was catalyzed by the work I did as a graduate student, analyzing mathematical models of HIV and the immune system. As a mathematician I found virtually every model I studied to be unrealistic. The biological assumptions on which the models were based varied from author to author, and this made no

---

16 http://www.mindfully.org/Health/2006/Why-I-Quit-HIV3mar06.htm

sense to me. It was around this time, too, that I became increasingly perplexed by the stories I heard about long-term survivors. From my admittedly inexpert viewpoint, the major thing they all had in common – other than HIV – was that they lived extremely healthy lifestyles. Part of me was becoming suspicious that being HIV positive didn't necessarily mean you would ever get AIDS.

Her conclusion was,

After ten years involved in the academic side of HIV research, as well as in the academic world at large, I truly believe that the blame for the universal, unconditional, faith-based acceptance of such a flawed theory falls squarely on the shoulders of those among us who have actively endorsed a completely unproved hypothesis in the interest of furthering our careers. Of course, hypotheses in science deserve to be studied, but no hypothesis should be accepted as fact before it is proven, particularly one whose blind acceptance has such dire consequences.... the craziness has gone on long enough. As humans – as honest academics and scientists – the only thing we can do is allow the truth to come to light.

So, the only thing my doctors could do now was to release me. In my eyes, they remained the same until the end – good AIDS specialists. "All those that have ceased medication will initially see an improvement, but after ten years they will have pneumonia, fever and things related," I heard my main doctor saying. Again the same speech? Yet he believed this, I could see it in his eyes, honest in his own truth. He had learned since the time he was a student of medicine that this is how things are, dictated by an international scientific consensus. In this circumstance, I would say only that this AIDS clergy had no imagination. They simply dictate the same sermon even if it has been greatly debunked. They are putting doctors and patients alike in a difficult position.

We played our roles again reluctantly. "Why are you taking such a risk Maria? All those who did came back to us shortly after and it was too late to save them," my second doctor informed me, and the same scenario was enacted. I had made my decision, there was no turning back. I telephoned another of my earlier AIDS doctors, the one who had so willingly helped me in London. I chose to reveal my emancipating decision and he responded no differently, "Why are you taking this risk Maria? Go to S. and he will explain it to you." These were the last farewells that had to be completed. I went to S.K. (we had become friends over the years, practically the same age) and he only asked me this, "So I should not try to persuade you?" "No, we are turning the page," I answered. He did not seem too disturbed by this. He only said, "Turning the page, eh?" Not too different from the conclusion of my primary doctor T.K., who had said "I am not going to persuade you and you are not going to persuade me. Good luck," and we shook hands.

Apparently they had been expecting this dramatic peak. Previously, when I went to the hospital to get my pills – the ones I discarded in the end – and I encountered S. K. in the hospital lobby, he would say: 'We love you, whatever you write' as if he felt almost betrayed. 'And I love you all, whatever I write,' I responded and we embraced. Our eyes were already saying "I'm sorry but we must part," after a twelve year relationship.

My withdrawal was not without forewarning. I gave them my books and my heart. I had invited them to the viewing of the documentary *"AIDS Inc."* and sent them a DVD of the documentary *"The Other Side of AIDS."* They should now be aware of the game being played at everyone's expense. Unless of course they threw them out in the garbage bin. What a divorce! A small misunderstanding, as they say.

As for the decisions taken by them on our behalf, Doctor Angelos Sicilian had the kindness to ask a friend and former AIDS specialist: "To begin with I told him I was not in the ball game and wanted to talk about white blood cells, which is my specialization. He suggested he show me all his evidence and combine it with mine. When he told me about his work on resistant viruses, I asked him who was responsible for isolating the HIV virus. I had now backed him into a corner. At first he said he sends his samples to England and it takes place there, and then he said it takes place in the United States because they have the patent for the procedure. In other words, he takes blood from Greece, sends it to his colleagues in England and they send it off to America! I expressed ever so gently my apprehension as to whether a reliable isolation is occuring. I mean, I do not know how it is possible for such a counterproductive, experimental process to be characterized as research. You cannot conduct an experiment and not monitor what goes on there!"

That doctor admitted by accident to where our blood samples are exported! The AIDS specialists simply execute their duties, and they do it with piety. My own doctor would attend the medical congresses religiously and educate himself so he could bring back the latest technology. Under the old routine, I would have been seeing them again in mid-July for my checkup with all the typical AIDS counts, like my T-4 cell count and my viral load count. These ceremonial blood tests performed by a team of doctors at eight in the morning were repeated every four months identically, incredibly monotonously, ungracefully and compulsorily. All were aware of the circumstance, the roles they played, the protagonists. There was no surprise in the forecast and yet we were all on edge. They had to monitor me forever from the moment I was found HIV positive. I felt like a convict who, after being released, had to appear at the local police station every few months to give blood. Over time the ceremonial blood test had been transformed into a friendly handshake between acquaintances, even though it hurt every time they failed for the thousandth time to find a vein to poke. I would receive the results in ten days. I always wondered why it took ten days to receive the results of a blood test. My question had now been answered. The blood is sent to the owners of our health (.!..) in America.

No, it would be best to never visit them again since I stopped the medication. Perhaps we could meet in another place if they wanted to appear useful for a fever, for example, or something transitory in the future. I asked again Dr Maniotis, after reassuring him that I was strong enough now. He replied:

> Dear Maria, I am pleased you are feeling so good. But do not expect to have the same disposition after meeting an AIDS specialist. I can say with certainty that you will be fine from here on out – as long as you stay far away from the doctors and their poisons. You need a homeopath or a naturopath who will help you remove the pharmaceutical toxins from your body so you can begin a new life and family with good health. Do not forget your regular walks when the sun is not too hot, because this is probably the safest way for your cells to regenerate. Simply walking assists in the reformation of marrow in the spinal cord which has been wounded by the bombardment of AIDS drugs for twelve years now.

That summer of 2007 passed like a dream. I could not believe how quickly I had returned to my former self. I felt the whole world had been granted to me. I said, "This summer I will remember forever." I could not believe how deeply I slept. "I have not slept like that in ten years" I said suddenly one morning. Of course, I could not get enough sleep. However even my awake hours were different. I did everything with zeal, and enjoyed my daily achievements.

At our holiday home, at one of the beaches in Attika, Gilles and I would apply the directions of Dr. Maniotis. Daily walks on the sand, the rocks and the pavement.

I would also spend endless hours on the computer. No one believed it, but that's where most of my self healing took place. "Unglue yourself from the computer, it will harm you," my brother would say. Yet I was untouchable next to my machine. I laughed, doubted, got secretly angry, and sometimes I would be overwhelmed by the thankful emails that came via my beloved web page. Only Gilles showed understanding of my idiosyncrasies. I had to make it to the end of my revelations to reclaim my life again in the outside world. There was no other way. I was riding a horse at full gallop, a true feeling of freedom.

In July 2007, before my first meeting with the homeopathic doctor, I felt I was being watched by many people but was now standing on solid ground. I had new allies and my frequently updated website (HIVwave.gr) was now, I felt, a reliable alternative source of health information for all worried about 'AIDS.'

5. A new universe of doctors

My first appointment with a renowned homeopath, in the Maroussi area of Athens, was finally arranged at the end of July, three months after stopping the AIDS pills. I kept on putting it off as I was already feeling good. I didn't know what to expect, he was the first of his kind that I would meet. The doctor, who did not look anything like a doctor, was waiting for us in an office so empty, so simple. No computer in sight, a picture on the wall, a vase, a smooth, crispy white doctor's coat hanging up behind the door, only some papers and one pencil in hand; it looked like he was there accidentally. I was not used to this.

I watched him write while I was talking, and he reminded me of a district schoolteacher. Just as I was wondering where he was taking the discussion, his questions took me by surprise. Chit-chat to chit-chat, it seemed as though he could guess what my problems were just by telling him a bit about myself.

He was less interested by the problem than the way I had handled it. What kind of person I was.....He suggested working on the vital energy of my system, and I liked the idea. I didn't mind the 100 euros for this visit, even though they didn't connect to the anti-star character of the man. The medicine he prescribed for me left me even more astounded. It was an extract from a seashell that would cost around 12 euros. From AZT, we were going on to seashells!

I would verify with Andy. His answer came back the same day, it was my message with his comments in capital letters:

> Saturday 21 July 2007
> Dear Andy
> We just got back from the homeopath.
> TERRIFIC!
> After being informed on my case, he said he could contribute to the reinforcement of my body power, especially when I plan to have a baby.
> THIS IS A TRUE STATEMENT.
> The hot/cold regimen is a good technique but he would suggest some homeopathic treatment, to reinforce my organism with the energy it needs most. That would be with non-chemical drugs, coming from the nature. Actually they are not commercial, they are prepared into capsules – diluting the natural essence in water – in homeopathic shops.
>
> YES – YOU NEED MICRONUTRIENTS BECAUSE YOU HAVE BEEN MALNOURISHED FOR A LONG TIME, AND HERBALS CAN HELP.
> After having collected information about my pathology, physiology, psychology and character, he decided what the homeopathic drug to prescribe: with the latin name Calcarea carbonica, it was prepared from oyster shells.
> I HAVEN'T HEARD OF IT-BUT WILL LOOK INTO IT.
> So, he prescribed for the first month Calcarea carbonica 1 x 100, one per day, first thing in the morning 15 minutes before breakfast, for the next 25 days Calcarea carbonica 1 x 10, one per day, the same way, until we meet again. Next appointment on September 18. It was the next empty space in his timetable, considering that August is a month off for all doctors. Usually he examines the impact of his therapy every month.
> THIS IS GOOD. STICK WITH IT!
> What do you thing of the homeopath' s sayings?

I THINK THEY ARE ALL SOUND AND WORTHY OF TRYING.

So glad to know you are with me

AND YOU WITH US!

ANDY

P.S. Calcarea carbonica.

Description

Calcarea carbonica, abbreviated as Calcarea carb., is a homeopathic remedy made from the middle layer of shells. In chemical terms, Calcarea carbonica is impure calcium carbonate, $CaCO_3$. Unlike most homeopathic remedies, which are made from substances soluble in water or alcohol, Calcarea carbonica must be prepared by a process called trituration.

Triturated material is ground or pounded until it is reduced to a fine powder. According to one homeopath, the discovery of trituration is a tribute to the genius of Samuel Hahnemann, the founder of homeopathy. "His method of preparing insoluble substances brought to light in this instance a whole world of therapeutic power formerly unknown."

General Use

Calcarea carbonica is a remedy that is given more frequently in so-called constitutional prescribing than to treat acute conditions. In constitutional prescribing, the homeopathic practitioner selects a remedy to treat the patient's complete symptomatology, based on a careful evaluation of his or her overall health. In homeopathy, constitution includes a person's heredity and life history as well as present lifestyle, environment, and medical history in the narrow sense.

Constitutional treatment is based on the assumption that chronic or recurrent illnesses reflect a specific weakness or vulnerability in the patient's total constitution. It is intended to stimulate healing at the deepest levels of the person's emotions and psyche as well as physical characteristics...

The note carried on. I went straight to the end: No side-effects, no interactions with other substances. Great! I would take it. That homeopathic medicine is supposed to stimulate healing, but would it work for me?

Could I trust that specific doctor? I thought about also asking X, who was the first to e-mail me about the benefits of homeopathy. He had proven to be good prophet so far. " If he prescribes only one drug each time, he is reliable", "X" expressed in a spartan way. I did not distinguish much enthusiasm in that answer. However, there was a complementary e-mail: "Basic Homeopathy is based on prescribing one medication which carries the strongest resemblance to the symptomatology of the patient, at the physical and psychological level. That is the reason why the patient gives the doctor a detailed mini-interview on the first visit". Besides homeopaths don't give out medication based on the illness of the patient, but on the consistency of the patient's character. For the same illness, they would give Gilles a different prescription.

The result of that treatment would still remain ambiguous. Was it the medication given to me by the homeopath that made me feel better each day or was it the absence of the drugs? Later I would learn more about the homeopathic treatments.

6. My former medical records:

My anger toward the medical establishment would subside at some point, as the need to find out how all this happened to me was growing everyday. I went and obtained my medical records ten months after stopping the AIDS therapy.

At the Laiko Hospital, the Archive Department did not keep the records of AIDS patients, they stay in the office of Dr. T.K. We are not included with the ill patients at the hospital nor with the healthy in the outside world, we belong to the kingdom of AIDS. I found an employee at the reception desk of the Archive Department and asked her to locate my records and the response was that she could do nothing. I would have to ask Dr. T.K. "Is it possible for you to ask?" beginning to feel restless and resistant, "But I don't want to." "But I cannot." It was impossible to decide which one of us would go. Until a miracle happened. "Oh, look, it's the director of the archives! She will explain everything," the employee cried out. Ms. Skomopoulou came forth and instantly knew what I wanted. "I know this girl, she is making quite a struggle, I have seen her on television. I will go myself to Dr. K.," she said and I wanted to kiss her. I completed the form and departed immediately. Two or three days later Ms. Skomopoulou called my home to inform me that my copies were ready.

We invited Dr. Angelos Sicilian to our home to review my records. We had noticed that they did not include the examinations that I had underwent and their results. What we had was only the evaluation of them done by the doctor, and not even in detail. "I will explain to you why this happens," said Dr. Sicilian. "When you have the medical records of a patient that was hospitalized, the results of the examinations end up in the office of the corresponding doctor whose job is to make a summary of the findings.

The x-rays were not included, only comments. The same with the results from the laboratory exams: only those details were recorded that were considered significant. So when you request your records you will not receive all the data but only those given by the office of the doctor in charge. Of course the complete file exists somewhere, they are not thrown into the garbage. But you are given no more than the comments from the relevant doctor. Perhaps there is useful information in the facts they excluded? "We see here a diagnosis of pneumonia but no explanation of the method used to diagnose it."

So, I was diagnosed with an illness of AIDS (Pneumocystis carini), although it was only a possibility, as my own doctor (T.K.) wrote in his medical notes. Our new doctor commented now: "The lies being told about the pathogenesis of HIV are innumerable and very dangerous." "There is only one unsigned chapter in my Pathology Anatomy book and it is the chapter on AIDS, where I found such lies that with the knowledge I have acquired these days it is now obvious to me. Two months prior I was unaware that the virus had never been found and thus I would have easily believed the part by the anonymous editor that the virus was detected in lymph nodes. It is also a mistake to explain the side-effects of the medication as part of the pathology. You were not lied to. They believed that. And it is not wise to dispute other people's beliefs."

My medical record gives a chest X-ray as the basis for the presumptive diagnosis of PCP, for which I started on Septrin (2 tablets per day) and AZT (500 mg/day). On the 15th day of treatment, I developed a fine maculopapular rash all over the body and face, an allergic reaction to Septrin, so it was discontinued. I was then given antihistamine tablets for the allergy, and Fansidar, which had previously been shown to prevent re-occurence of pneumocystis carinii pneumonia infections. In retrospect, if I really had a PCP problem, Septrin took care of it; the AZT given to fight 'HIV' was not required.

Angelos Sicilian was not sure at all that I had really suffered pneumonia: "In Greece pneumocystis carinii pneumonia (PCP) is uncommon. It is very rare, although AIDS patients are often wrongly diagnosed with it. I have not been taught the diagnosis of this illness and it was not been mentioned in any of the labs I have worked in. A research paper from the Evangelismos and Syngrou Hospitals does not refer to a single case of it, despite it's subject being its prevention. In other words, not one case has been diagnosed. In another research paper, PCP in an Immunocompetent Host, only one case is mentioned. It is very difficult to make this diagnosis for various reasons. No one has the expertise. If perhaps one of those experts, despite trying to fill in the voids made by others, is unable to identify the microbe, then, in my opinion, in practice he will simply play the role of God. He must maintain his reputation. He is not allowed to say: "I don't know." Moreover, there aren't many who can dispute his claim. He is on his own. Certainly he will score and win since he has no opponent."

"I am aware of this logic, as far as identification of bacteria goes in microbiology. Usually they produce hypothetical diagnoses. This is how we learn from the experts. My professor at the Hospital NIMTS was a military doctor and did not work like that. He struggled until the end to make an accurate identification. I avoid hypothetical diagnoses. I will refer to it as Gram Positive Grain, a general morphological term instead of a specific microbe. I have been scolded by everyone for this. I cannot teach my students to be exact because that is a poor teaching technique. This is how I have learned and have been criticized for paying attention to such detail. I do not know what can be done. If you were sick for months due to the antiretroviral treatment then it is possible you got, not only pneumocystis, but a host of other illnesses. However if the first diagnosis was pneumocystis and you had not taken earlier the antiretroviral drugs, as happened when you were first diagnosed, it is my understanding from your bio that they most likely invented your diagnosis."

That is why they could not detect it at the Athens Medical Center. You must be an AIDS specialist to diagnose it! They try to be correct with the wording. Dr. K. wrote about me "30/12/1995 - 16/01/1996, prolonged fever, possibly

PCR, anaemia." Possible pneumocystis carini, unsure; how this ambivalence influenced the rest of the situation is unknown.

Cytomegalovirus and tuberculosis meningitis were diagnosed for me later. Were these diagnoses also as tentative?

"CMV retinitis means a retinal infection from cytomegalovirus (CMV) and it was a false diagnosis because it was not based on a diagnosis of antibodies but simply on an ophthalmoscopy. This is improper," Dr Sicilian stated. "An ophthalmoscopy is insufficient to document viral causation. We can thus assume that the threatened loss of eyesight in you case, and others, was brought about by the drugs you were taking. In these papers the writers accept that retinitis from cytomegalovirus is caused by the medication as a side-effect. They refer to it elegantly as "the restoration of immune competence." There is no evidence you had such an illness. Now, as far as the tuberculous meningitis is concerned, I need more evidence. I do not believe it was tuberculosis. To find 5-7 acid resistant microbes, to see red coloured specks instead of blue after a process called the Ziehl-Nielsen colouring does not indicate tuberculosis when the culture is barren. Thus it was 'possibly' tuberculous meningitis".

On the positive side, Dr. K. presented clearly the reasoning behind his conclusions in his communications with the doctors in England about my case. They were exchanging views, something quite rare in the medical world. "Doctors usually do not take pleasure in cooperating with different specializations within the Greek framework. Those who come from outside the country are often better at this but the Greek mentality obstructs their efforts, no matter how good they may be;" our friend now informed us.

From that point of view, the correspondence between Dr. K. and Dr. R.H. in England, as seen in my medical file, was impressive. In one of these he stated: "Conclusions: Maria is an unfortunate female patient of ours who has developed a lot of HIV disease complications, mainly focused on the CNS (Central Nervous System). As I have mentioned in one of my previous e-mails, I am not very optimistic about her long term prognosis, although her family believes that those lesions might be curable. Surprisingly, her laboratory investigations are in contrast with the disease progression". Surprising indeed! When I visited London, the doctors expected to see me arriving on a stretcher but I was sill walking. His comment about the laboratory investigations suggests that a microbe or virus had not been found to cause the "disease progression;" thus the toxic effects of the 'AIDS' medication should have been suspected.

However Dr. Sicilian wanted to make something else clear. "I no longer have any doubt abut why I am doing all this. The answer is clear. Something horrible is occurring and we have to act accordingly. What makes me uneasy is that we might head in the wrong direction. Let's examine the facts we already have. First, Dr. K. accepts in his report that the diagnosis of pneumocystis carinii pneumonia is 'possible' and in my opinion that means laboratory confirmation never took place, just some x-rays. Second, I have not encountered to this day any man or woman in Greece who is in a position to verify with research a case of pneumocystis carinii pneumonia. Naturally there are several hospitals that I do not have access to and therefore cannot have knowledge of what goes on there. Third, we have some instances of Greek scientists who are giving diagnoses of probable pneumocystis carinii pneumonia. The reason is if someone has HIV, then every case of pneumonia must also be carinii. In other words, we all know the cards have been dealt and pneumocystis carinii pneumonia is the standard. Who can dispute this? How can we accuse anyone specifically when there is such a consensus amongst them? Can they all be punished? Or should just a few be punished instead? IT IS IMPORTANT TO ME THAT THE ACT IS CONDEMNED, NOT THE PERSON."

All that remained for us to do with the copies of my medical records we possessed was to review the fluctuation of the CD4 cells, as they were recorded every four months. There was a general satisfaction with my progress and the doctors attributed this to the good results of the drugs on my body.

Dr. Sicilian told us: "At the Centre of Disease Control and Prevention in the United States, efforts are apparently made to seduce the public by presenting the natural return of lymph cells after an infection as a therapeutic bodily response to the drugs … I will give you an example from your own history. Your first CD4 cell count at the hospital, when you were told you had pneumonia, was very low. This is quite common with these types of phenomena. I often see lymphocytes drop in number, especially in young people with pneumonias. The impressive part is that one finds this in older people too. However, in young folks one can observe within one afternoon a change in lymphocyte numbers. They may begin to increase. A drop in lymphocyte numbers is by no means due to the deaths of lymphocytes. On the contrary it means a transient shift of many of them to places in need of defence. Usually it means they have gone into some lymph nodes for 'conferences' and an 'exchange of information.' Following the conferences, the lymphocytes may increase rapidly in the blood either due to a sudden movement of them or because of the creation of more of them. They multiply for specific purposes. My conclusion is that the AIDS researchers interpret this natural transient drop in lymphocyte numbers as due to them dying, while this is really not occurring. When the cells begin increasing in number, they wrongly credit this to the therapy. This is why the confession of my AIDS specialist friend is so vital, that even in those not taking medication the same increase in lymphocyte numbers is observed in the blood."

Our new doctor had yet more suspicions. "The percentages of lymphocytes are missing [in the medical file]. I have yet to witness this kind of medical analysis. They provide only the number of CD4 cells, and not the total number of lymphocytes which includes the CD4 cells. This is the first time I have seen this." "Why is the CD4 examination done only to HIV positives? I do not know of anyone else who has done it," I added with my own doubt. "It seems odd to you?" "Yes, very." "It is peculiar and curious because even we are not allowed to learn why such an important test does not exist in public research centers. Here there is something cunning going on as the equipment has become more expensive purposefully. Whatever they want, they either increase or lower the price. The same is happening with the research involved with HIV. As a microbiologist for years I have heard much about the CD4 count and yet have never witnessed it happening anywhere. It is possible only in a few hospitals. I ask myself, when you have the same equipment for years it is logical for prices and costs to fall. This occurs with all equipment and new technology. I do not understand why the new equipment that examines the CD4 cells is not shared so that doctors everywhere can learn by using it. I would like to delve into this topic."

Gilles did his own Google search and found an electronic picture of a CD4 molecule[17]. It had been discovered in the 1970's and earned the name CD4 in 1984. What a coincidence, the same year as the HIV proclamation! CD4 means Cluster of Differentiation 4. CD4 tests count the number of T cells containing the CD4 receptor, they are considered critical in assessing the immune system of 'AIDS' patients.

"I know what it is but I have never seen it in the laboratory. I use only the known blood related analyses that show the total number of lymphocytes. I have not seen how CD4 cells are separated from lymphocytes. I do not know, it may sound like a conspiracy theory, but it is very difficult to conduct any research with this equipment in Greece and I presume in many other places. It is used mainly for AIDS work".

As far as the viral load in my blood is concerned, it was considered "undetectable" in my last blood counts. I never understood what that meant, how could they count the viral load of a virus that cannot be detected, even with the HIV tests? "The so-called viral load is based upon the PCR technology and some believe that when this test exhibits positive results that is evidence of HIV. Perhaps it is enough to listen to a statement by Kary Mullis who won the Nobel Prize in 1993 for his discovery of the PCR method. As the person who made the discovery he refutes the claim that the method detects the presence of that specific virus".

However, the AIDS establishment does not bow to anyone. Instead of withdrawing discreetly after the reaction of the Nobel-winning professor, they kept using his invention to reinforce their claims to have discovered the HIV virus. We of course never learned in the mainstream media of Kary Mullis' statement that his invention is utterly unable to detect HIV.

Behold now the history of antiretroviral therapy that I took as a result of this affair. I found a reference made by Dr. T.K. to Dr. R.H. in London, showing that from the 10th of March, 1995, I began taking AZT. From the 23rd of November 1995 until the 24th of September 1996, I took AZT and Hivid. From the 25th of September 1996 until the 26th of May 1999, I took the first Protease Inhibitor (PI) drug cocktail consisting of Norvir, Hivid and 3TC. From the 27th of May 1999 until January 2005, I took Crivixan, Hivid and 3TC.

Finally, from January 2005 until stopping the 'AIDS' treatment on the 23rd of April 2007, I took Stocrin, Emtriva and Viread. These are their commercial names.

Disconcertingly, I recently learnt that the sale and distribution of Hivid was

---

17 Wikipedia, cd4 page, last viewed June 14 2008.

discontinued at the end of 2006, yet this was the drug I took eight out of the ten years of the therapy. The most recent treatment guidelines state that HIVID should NOT be administered in combination with AZT or 3TC. This is in the M.D./Alert[18] sent to warn doctors by its manufacturer, Roche Pharmaceuticals.

For their true value, not a word. There is no indication that those drugs fight any virus at all, as Dr. Maniotis said in an interview with the Greek reporter Lambros Papantoniou[19]. The antiretroviral medication can have an antibiotic effect and kill bacteria, mycoplasma and fungi that may appear in an immunodeficiency patient. In long-term use, they weaken the immune system and other organs. Sooner or later, the whole organism becomes vulnerable.

We can now understand what happened in my circumstance. During the 'AIDS' treatment period, changing the medication relieved me each time from the serious adverse effects of the previous prescription. I was saved from severe neurological damages with the latest medication cocktail, only because it replaced a more toxic combination that is now proscribed.

---

18   HIVID (zalcitabine) tablets. Dear Health Care Professional Letter. (June 2006),
     http://www.fda.gov/cder/drug/shortages/Roche_HIVID_MDLetter.pdf
19   AIDS, a Global Scandal. "Paraskevi+13", December 7, 2007

Chapter 5

Big Brother: Total supervision by the AIDS establishment

1. Salvation is called dissent

Should I remain silent after I was saved from AIDS? Probably I should hide even more. "You are dangerous" I heard for the first time in my life after I decided to start questioning my HIV diagnosis. It was by someone anonymous. As long as I kept hiding I had been no problem for the others, so what was different now?

I have been in the sights of thousands of malevolent people ever since I made an appearance as the HIV-positive Maria K. on the Internet, New Year's Eve 2006. Maybe I had caused the rage myself by naming my first book *How I defeated AIDS?*[20] I didn't know it was forbidden to do so. And how did I conquer it? It was quite simple. I discovered that they are lying! Something like that meant to me the beginning of their end: People in whom I had believed for so long; whoever they were, they were lying, consciously or unwittingly!

In the beginning the scientists were saying that "the virus is only transmitted through blood and semen." That had saved my sanity for many of those years, as it meant I was not a killing machine if I had sex. Although I could no longer locate that information, it turned out to be right. I could not find my equivalent in the opposite sex anywhere; and none of my beloved partners, after my positive diagnosis, was found to be positive. That's how the provocative question in the first version of my website occurred: "If there is an HIV-positive heterosexual male, write to me, anonymously if you want".

I wanted to let others know that someone is playing with our health and mind. Many people agreed, however some opposed me, finding it impossible to believe that most scientists around the world are wrong. But I had started to find many other prestigious scientists around the world who questioned the conventional wisdom. I thought that those revelations would trouble everyone. However, I was attacked by many who said: "I am conscienceless, an opportunist, hypocrite, mischievous, dangerous to my fellow citizens, HIV-positive or not, young or old, mothers, husbands and children. "

In the first days, I was left wonder-struck. Wounded. However, those strange anonymous citizens made me dig even more into the hidden scenery behind the AIDS concept, to understand their problem. I could have stayed in the virgin

---

20 Πώς νίκησα το AIDS, Kastaniotis editor, 2006. Available only in Greek.

stage of revelations with the "*How I conquered AIDS*" book, if they had treated me well. But they ran after me. Pushing me more into the comforting arms of Gilles, the knight of the Internet who would later become my husband. "Don't pay any attention to them, be prepared for such behaviour from now on", he had written to me from the start.

My second book, *The love game in the time of AIDS,* [21] exposed more evidence about the AIDS deception, as I had uncovered it so far. The book received a positive review in the Greek magazine *Zenith.* However, the AIDS orthodoxy had been overcome by frenzy and they reacted effectively this time – their second mistake, for it made me angry. I blame on them the fact that it has not been reviewed anywhere in the mainstream press. It even influenced my book launch. The publisher asked me quite mysteriously to find representatives from both sides of the field of AIDS to speak about the book.

He did not have that requirement for my first book. "It is like writing a new testimony for the Armenian genocide and you are requested to find a Turkish official to present your book", commented a seropositive friend of mine, who published her first autobiography last year, available only in Greek: "*Of course you are not concerned*", using the nickname Alexandra Athinaiou.

There was nothing left to do, but to go even further. They wouldn't stop attacking me, but Gilles showed me the way around that.

More and more I would learn interesting things, such as how the 'science' of AIDS gained predominance over time. Billions of dollars were available for 'AIDS' research, but only if it focused on reinforcing the HIV/AIDS dogma. Thus those subsidized studies spread like a wildfire, increasing the "corpus" of scientific consensus, as it is called. However, it is strange that, despite more than 100,000 studies being carried out so far, nowhere can we find a proof that HIV causes AIDS, or that it is infectious, or even that it is a sexually transmitted disease.

What happens if you ask for the specific scientific references that prove HIV causes AIDS? In the words of Nobel laureate Kary Mullis, as recorded in the "*AIDS inc.*" (2007) documentary by Gary Null:

> AIDS researchers now are getting neurotic if you ask them any questions. There was a time when I first started asking questions. All I wanted to know was, 'Where are the papers?', 'Just tell me the papers that you read that convinced you that HIV is the cause of AIDS because I need to reference those papers' – I was working on a test for HIV with PCR, and I needed to write a little report to the NIH and say here's the progress we've made. And the first line of it was, 'HIV is the probable cause of AIDS', and I thought that was true before I got into it and involved. I said, 'Where's the reference for that quote?' And I looked for it for about two or three years and I never did find it. And by the end of two years, I'd asked everybody at every meeting that

---

21 Το παιχνίδι του έρωτα στα χρόνια του AIDS, Kastaniotis editor, 2006. Available only in Greek.

I had gone to that talked about AIDS. I'd ask, you know, everyone – I'd look through every computer database. There is no reference. There is nobody who should get credit for that statement. Now that's a pretty weird situation in science where getting credit for a discovery is the most important thing in your life as a scientist.

A part of the explanation for that bizarre reality was given by David Rasnick (PhD), also in the documentary *AIDS Inc.*:

> Those that control and maintain the HIV hypothesis of AIDS are two basic institutions: The Centers for Disease Control (CDC), and the National Institutes of Health in Bethesda, Maryland. It will probably come as a surprise to the public to learn that they are military organizations. When you have these military structures in the CDC and the National Institutes of Health, you can control the debate. You can control the information flow. Not only that, since the National Institutes of Health is the primary source of funding for all academic medical scientific research, they can control who gets funding to do what research. And in that fashion they can control what gets published, and more importantly what you exclude.

Who may benefit from the AIDS deception? In the book *State of Fear* (2004), Michael Crichton explains it well: "the military-industrial complex is no longer the primary driver of society [...] For the last 15 years we have been under the control of an entirely new complex, far more powerful and far more pervasive. I call it the politico-legal-media complex [...] And it is dedicated to promoting fear in the population, under the guise of promoting safety."

That still could not justify so much passion against someone who has won her fight against AIDS and does not hide it. It took me some time to understand why I was considered so dangerous. The whole campaign, financed in large parts by public money, is based on an unsupported hypothesis, that the virus HIV cause AIDS. That was hazardous from the beginning. If people start to look into it and discover that their tax money is wasted on such false premises, they will stop supporting its funding and blame those who mislead them. If HIV does not cause AIDS, how many people have died up until now, because of false diagnosis? And how many have been imprisoned as killers simply for making love?

2. Scientific careers are threatened

In 1987[22] Dr. Peter Duesberg, the outstanding expert on retroviruses, stated that these could not cause the AIDS problem. But, instead of presenting an adequate rebuttal, the AIDS orthodoxy managed to damage his career by not

---

22 P. Duesberg, "Retroviruses as carcinogens and pathogens: Expectations and reality," Cancer Research 47, 1199 (1987).

renewing his research grants, stopping him from publishing in prestigious scientific journals, and even scaring away graduate students.

As I learned that numerous careers had been destroyed and the culprits never punished, I started to worry about my new friends. I did not have to worry about my own career at that point, I was only beginning to discover a hidden facet of our reality, to understand the more complex picture and what was happening behind the scenes.

I was wondering about Dr Andrew Maniotis, how was it possible for him to remain in his position and challenge the dogma, while Dr. Peter Duesberg had been given such a hard time. Although voices of dissent have become more widespread nowadays, those who dare express their dissent still put their career at risk, because it affects a very powerful establishment.

On September 13 2007, a dark cloud appeared. Andy had sent an e- mail to Lambros, who forwarded it to me. Something was going on. Obviously, the first one didn't want to make me anxious with every detail of the conflict, but the second one intended to keep me informed. Andy wrote:

> Dear Lambros,
> I don't know what has happened yet. I stayed home, my boss took off for the next several days, there supposedly were some high level meetings today. I don't know if I still have a job there.
> Wainberg, and about 10 others are doing the same thing to Rebecca Culshaw,[23] asking the University President and administration to fire her. She was the one who wrote that piece you liked so much and that Maria translated. She and I are going to work together, and perhaps get other professors and respected scientists to write letters of support to the same people that Wainberg, and his brownshirts wrote to. But nothing is happening yet.
> I very much appreciate all of your support and friendship at this time, because you give me courage when I need it.
> You are a remarkable human being, Lambros.
> Yasu,
> Andreas

This letter of support from Stephen Davis presents a clear picture of some of his attackers from the 'AIDS' establishment:

> To: B. Joseph White, President
> University of Illinois, Chicago
> 414 Administrative Office Building, MC-760
> 1737 W. Polk St
> Chicago IL

---

23 Rebecca Culshaw, author of the book "*Science sold Out: Does HIV Really Cause AIDS?*" was teaching at the University of Texas.

Dear President White,

As a former Arizona state senator (32nd Arizona Legislature), I am writing on behalf of Dr. Maniotis, having been sent a copy of a letter addressed to you from Mark Wainberg dated September 10, 2007 (enclosed below).

In that letter, Wainberg states that "Dr Maniotis has allied himself with those who question whether HIV causes AIDS in the first place" as if this were some kind of high crime. The fact is that science is supposed to be a process of questioning any and all theories, proving those that are true by experimental and experiential evidence, and discarding those that turn out to be false.

Having personally read and researched over 1500 scientific studies, research documents and articles in peer-reviewed journals, I am convinced there is a serious question that should be addressed concerning the cause(s) of AIDS and the role of HIV in this deadly disease. I am proud to be counted among those who raise those questions based on the lack of scientific evidence supporting HIV as the cause of AIDS; and Dr. Maniotis is only one of more than 2300 researchers, scientists, doctors and other health care professionals who have had the courage to publicly express similar concerns - including two Nobel Prize winners in chemistry and medicine, and members of the U.S. National Academy of Sciences (There is a list of many on www.rethinkingaids.com).

The indisputable fact is that HIV fails every scientific test to be called the cause of AIDS, including Koch's Postulates, Farr's Law, the first epidemiological law of viral and microbial diseases, cluster formations, and even the definition of the word 'infectious' itself – tried and true criteria that have been in use in medical research for decades, but are now discarded to support the theory that HIV=AIDS. Dr. Maniotis is to be commended, not punished, for standing up and asking the tough questions to try to find the truth behind this terrible tragedy.

Wainberg also claims that Dr. Maniotis "has seriously libeled Dr. Robert Gallo, a scientist who is credited with the discovery of HIV." First of all, Dr. Gallo is, at best, a co-discoverer of HIV, along with Dr. Luc Montagnier at the Pasteur Institute in Paris, France. Dr. Gallo, in fact, tried to steal a retrovirus discovered by Montagnier in 1983 called LAV and claim it was his own discovery called HTLV-III, taking credit for this "discovery" at a press conference on April 23, 1984. He was later caught in the act, and only after intense international negotiations, culminating in an agreement signed by President Ronald Reagan then-Prime Minister Jacque Chirac, did France agree not to sue Gallo and the U.S. in international court for this scientific fraud and agreed to call Gallo a "co-discoverer" of the retrovirus later named HIV in exchange for sharing in the royalty payments. All of this is part of public record.

However, since I am not privy to everything Dr. Maniotis has said about Dr. Gallo, I can only suggest that you do your own research about the life and times of Dr. Robert Gallo, his record of scientific misconduct, his lies (most notably on his patent application for the so-called HIV tests), his theft of other people's work (such as another retrovirus discovered by a Japanese team), and similar outrageous behavior. One virologist went so far as to call Gallo "a scientific gangster" "who could not be trusted to tell the time correctly". So I would question whether Dr. Maniotis actually "libeled" Dr. Gallo, or whether he simply told the truth about this man's checkered past.

(For more information about Dr. Gallo, I refer you to the investigations of Gallo by the Office of Scientific Integrity of the National Institutes of Health (1991), the Office of Research Integrity of the Department of Health and Human Services (1992), and the Subcommittee on Oversight and Investigations of the U.S. House of Representatives, 1994, among others.)

I realize that the prevailing opinion at this time is that HIV causes AIDS. However, at other times the prevailing opinion has been that the earth was flat and the center of the universe around which the sun and other planets revolved. I think the University of Illinois, Chicago, should be proud to have Dr. Maniotis as a member of its faculty, and I predict that it will not take too many more years for the rest of the scientific community to recognize the validity of his questions. In fact, the most recent research (again, published in peer-reviewed scientific journals) is already proving to be right, i.e.:

Viral load measurements failed in 90% of the cases in predicting the loss of CD4 cells, which HIV is supposed to destroy. In fact, viral load tests were only able to predict "progression to disease" in 4% to 6% of the HIV-Positives studied. This study concludes that there must be "nonvirological mechanisms as the predominant cause of CD4 cell loss" (Rodriguez et al, Journal of the American Medical Association (JAMA), September 27, 2006).

"Our new interdisciplinary research has thrown serious doubt on one popular theory of how HIV affects these [CD4] cells" (New Scientist, May 2007).

"Grade 4 Events are as important as AIDS events in the era of HAART." In other words, more people in the U.S. are dying from the side-effects of the anti-retroviral medications than are dying from HIV/AIDS-related illnesses. (Reisler et al, Journal of Acquired Immune Deficiency Syndrome, December 2003)

After more than twenty-five years and many billions of dollars, we still have no cure and no vaccine for AIDS. I thus find it entirely appropriate for Dr. Maniotis to ask: Is it because we have the wrong cause to begin with? And I find it admirable that the University of

Illinois, Chicago, would support the search for truth, no matter where it may lead.

As for Wainberg, you should know that he receives large sums of money from the very pharmaceutical companies who profit in the billions of dollars from the faulty HIV=AIDS hypothesis. (Wainberg has disclosed that he has received grant/research support from GlaxoSmithKline, Bristol-Myers Squibb, and Serono. He has also served as a consultant to and/or was on the advisory board for Pfizer, GlaxoSmithKline, Bristol-Myers Squibb, and Gilead Sciences, and has served on the speaker's bureau for GlaxoSmithKline, Gilead Sciences, Bristol-Myers Squibb, and ViroLogic. 24

When I served in the Senate, I was not permitted by law to vote or lobby on behalf of any legislation in which I had a financial interest. Not only does that make common sense; it makes ethical sense. In short, Wainberg's opinion is not objective, nor should it be trusted. Dr. Maniotis, on the other hand, has nothing to gain by asking his questions, except a quest for the truth. In fact, he has everything to lose. Furthermore, it is this same Wainberg who has been videotaped making such statements as: "As far as I'm concerned, those who attempt to dispel the notion that HIV is the cause of AIDS are perpetrators of death, and I, for one, would very much like to see the Constitution of the United States and similar countries have some means in place that we can charge people who are responsible for endangering public health with charges of endangerment and bring them up on trial..It strikes me that someone who would perpetrate the notion that HIV is not the cause of AIDS is perhaps motivated by sentiments of pure evil - that such a person may perhaps really want millions of people in Africa and elsewhere to become infected by this virus and go on to die of it.. I suggest to you that Peter Duesberg is perhaps the closest thing we have in this world to a scientific psychopath." (Dr. Peter Duesberg is a former California Scientist of the Year and a member of the U.S. National Academy of Sciences. Needless to say, Wainberg is not. Actual video available upon request.)

As for the letter from John Moore, which you also received, here is how one writer described Moore.. "He has never published any scientific paper about the origins of the AIDS pandemic. During the last decade or so, Moore has developed a reputation for writing witty and acerbic commentaries on all sorts of AIDS-related subjects, and in the process has become something of a media darling, quoted on a regular basis by several science journalists. However, many who work in the field of AIDS are skeptical about Moore, feeling that he has

---

24 Source: www.medscape.com/viewarticle/532151)

become carried away with his own reputation as an 'AIDS expert'."
Therefore, I hope you would seriously question the source of these
attacks on Dr. Maniotis, and ultimately ignore them, allowing Dr.
Maniotis to continue his true scientific inquiry, with even greater
support from UIC.

When Dr. Maniotis and his work are finally vindicated, I'm hopeful
that the University of Illinois, Chicago, will be at his side to share in
his success.

Sincerely,
Stephen Davis
P.S. I have cc'd those who received Wainberg's email.

There was a positive conclusion that time (he was not fired then, but the
lobbying continued and we later learned that his contract may not be renewed):

Dear Lambros,
I had the formal hearing with the dean(s) today... The meeting was
called to advise the president of the University, Joe White, what to do
in response to the letters against me. They said we could do nothing,
apologize to Wainberg, or, fire you. After I explained my side of the
story, they said,

"Wow! Then, when in future you write your criticisms of the AIDS
establishment, just make sure you don't do any ad hominem attacks on
people's character, and state your full title and rank. I thanked them,
and said, "I always have represented my true title, and I will continue
to not attack people's characters, and will, from now on, state my full
rank and title.

3. Journalists are restricted

I realized that most of us will not have an idea about all of this except if we
search on our own, as that information was restricted early on. I recently noticed
Dr. Peter Duesberg, who started questioning the HIV/AIDS theory in the `80s,
saying in the documentary" *AIDS Inc.":*
\

Reporters came. They asked questions and found my views and my
hypothesis very logical and convincing, but they never aired them
because they were censored at the highest level, presumably when an
executive producer would have called the National Institutes of Health
to ask: "Is this all right to show this view advanced by Duesberg from
Berkeley?"

Over twenty years, there where very few exceptions to the almost complete
censorship about AIDS dissent in the main press. We should thank the
courageous journalists, and their editors, who did not follow the orders of the
powerful AIDS establishment.

In 1992-1994, *The Sunday Times* (London) became the first, and only, national newspaper to run a series of articles presenting the other side of AIDS, written by its scientific editor, Neville Hodgkinson. It stopped when the editor of *The Sunday Times*, Andrew Neil, was replaced in 1994.

In 1996, Neville published the book *"AIDS: The Failure of Contemporary Science."*[25] He commented about the reaction of the other journalists, in the documentary *"AIDS Inc."* (2007):

> When I was first reporting on the views of scientists who challenged the HIV story, I really thought that my colleagues would be quick to pick up and look at this for themselves. I was amazed that, instead of doing that, they not only ignored the critique, but they actually attacked me and *The Sunday Times* for having raised these issues.

It took a long while before another mainstream publication with a large distribution would touch that issue. In March 2006, Celia Farber ("the most dangerous AIDS reporter"[26] according to the magazine for seropositive people *POZ*) published "Out of control: AIDS and the corruption of medical science"[27], a 15-page article in the venerable *Harper's* magazine.

Besides presenting the AIDS deception, it gave a concrete, shocking, example of how corporate and political influence led the "AIDS science" leaders in the USA (at the NIH) to approve the invalid results of clinical studies... using the very toxic nevirapine and AZT, "to prevent the transmission of HIV" from pregnant women to their children.

There was a very strong reaction from the AIDS establishment. Robert Gallo himself co-signed a document claiming[28] to show numerous errors in the *Harper's* magazine article, and a new website, "AIDStruth.org," was created to counter the criticism.

> In March 2006, after Harper's Magazine published a feature article by AIDS denialist Celia Farber, a number of scientists and activists joined together to create a website for the purpose of countering AIDS denialist misinformation and debunking denialist myths, while providing truthful information about HIV and AIDS. The result is the AIDSTruth.org website. [29]

---

25 N. Hodgkinson,*"AIDS: The Failure of Contemporary Science, How a Virus that Never Was Deceived the World"*, Fourth Estate Publishers U.K. 1996, 420 pages..

26 Interview Celia Farber, *The Most Dangerous AIDS Reporter*, by Richard Berkowitz, POZ April 2000

27 *Out of control: AIDS and the corruption of medical science*, by Celia Farber, Harper's Magazine, March 2006
   http://harpers.org/archive/2006/03/0080961 accessed August 22, 2008

28 Correcting Gallo: Rethinking AIDS Responds to Harper's 'Out of Control' Critics
   http://www.rethinkingaids.com/GalloRebuttal/overview.html

. 29 About AIDSTruth.org, http://www.aidstruth.org/new/about, accessed January 6, 2009.

Despite the attempts to counteract the impact of the revelations, in May 13, 2008, a Semmelweis Society International (SSI) "Clean Hands" Award was presented to Dr. Peter Duesberg and Celia Farber. After hostile attacks by AIDS fanatics, a private investigator and retired Los Angeles Police officer, Clark Baker, was hired by the SSI to investigate Duesberg and Farber. Baker's complete report, "Gallo's Egg",[30] vindicates those who expose the AIDS deception, and has been posted on many websites around the world. It describes how AIDS junk science is a criminal racket. Of course, the mainstream press covered neither the awards nor the report.

One explanation was given by Dr. Henry Bauer, Professor Emeritus of Chemistry at Virginia Polytechnic Institute, in his book *The Origins, Persistence and Failings of HIV/AIDS Theory* (2007):

> As science and technology have become more tightly interwoven and connected to industry and government and indeed to every sector of society, complex associations tend to form that function as research cartels and thereby effect knowledge monopolies. The media collude unwillingly: they do not practice skeptically investigative reporting about whatever scientific dogma happens to hold sway. In some ways the media are hapless, because they are not independent of those cartels. They depend on them for the information that is the basis of their livelihood. [...] But could the power of the purse strings and the interlocked organizations of science exert similarly strong regulation in open, free, democratic societies? The answer has to be "Yes", because there are concrete examples.

The concentration of media ownership made it easier from the start to reduce the expression of dissent. In 1983, at the beginning of the AIDS deception, 50 corporations controlled the vast majority of all news media in the U.S. At the time, Ben Bagdikian was called "alarmist" for pointing this out in his book, *The Media Monopoly*. In the 4th edition, published in 1992, he wrote, "in the U.S., fewer than two dozen of these extraordinary creatures own and operate 90% of the mass media" – controlling almost all of America's newspapers, magazines, TV and radio stations, books, records, movies, videos, wire services and photo agencies. He predicted then that eventually this number would fall to about half a dozen companies. This was greeted with skepticism at the time. When the 6th edition of *The Media Monopoly* was published in 2000, the number had fallen to six. Since then, there have been further mergers and the scope has expanded to include new media like the Internet market. More than 1 in 4 Internet users in the U.S. now log in with AOL Time-Warner, the world's largest media corporation.

In 2004, Bagdikian's revised and expanded book, *The New Media Monopoly*, shows that only 5 huge corporations –Time Warner, Disney, Murdoch's News Corporation, Bertelsmann of Germany, and Viacom (formerly CBS) – now

---

30 http://www.rethinkingaids.com/reference/GallosEgg-17Jul08.pdf

control most of the media industry in the U.S. and General Electric's NBC is a close sixth.

Those mega-corporations control what will be published in the USA. For instance, why did most of the U.S. media kept silent about the important news presented under the title "Threat of world Aids pandemic among heterosexuals is over, report admits", by *The Independent* (UK) newspaper in June 8, 2008[31] (the first two sentences quoted here)

> A quarter of a century after the outbreak of Aids, the World Health Organization (WHO) has accepted that the threat of a global heterosexual pandemic has disappeared.
>
> In the first official admission that the universal prevention strategy promoted by the major Aids organizations may have been misdirected, Kevin de Cock, the head of the WHO's department of HIV/Aids said there will be no generalized epidemic of Aids in the heterosexual population outside Africa.

So, the threat of a heterosexual AIDS pandemic is officially over and decades of predictions that AIDS would spread through general populations across the globe were wrong. That news quickly spread on the Internet all around the world. However, as confirmed by a Google search (in September 2008) for the quote "there will be no generalized epidemic of Aids in the heterosexual population." there was not even one article about that printed in the American mass media. That is called censorship.

I was thinking that in our country, Greece, we had been kept almost totally in the darkness. But again I was surprised to learn recently that there were voices in Athens who had formulated the "other side" of AIDS much earlier than me. A new friend of the website let me know that the specialized magazine *Trito Mati* had printed relevant articles in November 1998 (in Greek) *It will shock you, but fill you with hope: The terrible conspiracy of AIDS!* and in May 2004 *The AIDS fraud and the pharmaceutical cartel: An unpunished crime* by someone signing "Mithridates". I will only quote here [free translation] how he had described the background of the censorship:

> The attack on scientists who disagree and denounce the "official" hypothesis of HIV/AIDS, promoted by the pharma-cartel and its scientific representatives, is revelatory for the "scientism" of the latter: Deprived of the freedom to question mainstream views, refused permission to publish those questions in the standard journals of scientific research (i.e. *Nature, Lancet*) and, last but not least, ejected from positions of influence at universities and deprived of financing for research (i.e. in the cases of Duesberg and Stefan Lanka), followed by the FBI (Duesberg), having their moral integrity attacked and their

---

31 *"Threat of world Aids pandemic among heterosexuals is over, report admits"*, by Jeremy Laurance, 8 June 2008, The Independent (UK).

credibility dismissed in nosy gossip by complicit journalists – mercenaries of the cartel [...], and attempts of murder (in the case of professor Heinrich Kremer). [...] Dr. Robert E. Willner left Spain speechless after getting inoculated with the blood of Pedro Tocino, an HIV-positive hemophiliac. That demonstration, to prove that HIV virus does not cause AIDS and is really harmless (Willner would accept, the same as Duesberg, that the virus exists) made the front page news in every major newspaper of Spain, but that historical event was never mentioned in the American mass-media... Dr. Peter Duesberg has also offered to be inoculated by the HIV virus in order to pinpoint his opposition to the current AIDS dogma...

Some of the "dissidents" say that the virus exists? Peter Duesberg had explained back in 1992: *"now we have people arguing whether the virus that doesn't cause AIDS actually exists."*

Of course Mithridates was aware of that. I recently met him, a successful Athenian lawyer who was living with an 'HIV-positive' lady when he did his own research on AIDS and published it in probably the only magazine that was ready to accept it in Greece. The mass media again did not pick up the issue.

The ability to keep us in the dark, without us understanding that we suffer from extensive censorship, has been recognized as a new tool of fascism. It is not forbidden to tell the truth, but the lies are supported with such great subsidies that people find it almost impossible to understand what has happened from 1984 until now. Any attempt to express an objection is suppressed. "One of the best defenses of the AIDS establishment is telling you that it is far too complex for you to understand. You can't possibly understand it. Don't try. Just trust us. And that has been successful so far", I heard David Crowe, the director of the Alberta Reappraising AIDS Society saying in the *"AIDS Inc."* documentary. "At some point, and I hope it won't be in too distant future, we'll all be able looking back on AIDS and say 'How could we have been bamboozled for so long?'"

I think few in the media have spoken out so far, not even in private, because few of them know. I lived 18 happy years in the newspaper *"To Vima"*, actually it was my refuge, and I had never heard a whisper about the 'other side of AIDS'. No wonder the thought never occurred to me.

When I started discovering that alternative reality in 2006, and published my first book, everybody around was as amazed as me, they showed interest, they supported me. A year later, nothing would be the same, as if there had been a secret notification. It then became obvious that the climate which preserves the AIDS dogma all over the world also censors any attempt to pose disturbing questions about corruption in AIDS research, suppressing journalists who try to examine the views of the "dissidents", stopping discussions about the toxicity of the drugs and the resulting deaths. Often, a well-paid executive in the correct place is enough to stop anyone from expressing dissent about the HIV/AIDS dogma. Scientific critics of great esteem are called "denialists" while the paid "speakers" for the pharmaceutical industries are spoken of positively as "activists" and "researchers".

Personally, I continued to have a job with the support of people around me, as if nothing ever happened, as if no AIDS dissenters existed, as if there was no need to discuss it further.

The parallel evolution of the alternative press and the Internet has now created a space for communication where tight control is impossible in democratic countries. However, in this information war, we should be aware that alternative media can also be manipulated, and used, sometimes unwittingly, to spread disinformation. Thus, the majority of those relying on alternative publications still remain ignorant about such major issues as the AIDS deception.

Nevertheless, as the awareness expands, it will become harder to continue fooling us.

4. The corruption of medical practice

We are prevented from fully trusting doctors when we learn that medical procedures frequently have been corrupted. A large-scale example of this corruption was reported by the *Greek American Weekly Newspaper*, one of those independent newspapers that says things as they are.[32] The following is an excerpt in a free translation from Greek.

> America pharmaceutical companies and doctors are over the moon as they earn millions of dollars with the 'spread' of HIV/AIDS, on the back of innocent people who are sick, although it is not yet clear if the so-called HIV virus, if it exists, causes AIDS – the collapse of the immunity system – or if this is something else that has occurred throughout human history. The American Government is involved in this hoax (because that is what it's all about) since it has approved all the drugs that are on the market to deal with AIDS, drugs similar to those used as chemotherapies against cancer. This medication itself can cause AIDS diseases, and ultimately kill the patients. [...]
>
> The state of Minnesota voted in a law that obliges the pharmaceutical companies to provide records of all payments given to health care professionals to encourage the prescription of their drugs ... A major state inquiry showed that from 1997 to 2006, according to the

---

32 Πλουτίζουν σε βάρος των ασθενών με AIDS, Greek News, April 2, 2007.
   http://www.greeknewsonline.com/modules.php?name=News&file=article&sid=6524
   , accessed January 2009.

   Most of the statistics presented can be verified in The New York Times article
   "Doctors' Ties to Drug Makers Are Put on Close View", by Gardiner Harris and
   Janet Roberts, March 21, 2007
      http://www.nytimes.com/2007/03/21/us/21drug.html, accessed January 2009.

files of the pharmaceutical companies, 5,500 doctors, nurses and others who were supposed to focus on treating sick people, got away with receiving 57 million dollars under the table from the drug manufacturers!!!

Another 40 million dollars were donated to clinics, research centers and other organizations, to promote some pseudo-diagnostics. We are talking about such a big hoax that the world has never come across such before. More than 20 % of the doctors in the state have grabbed illegal money for achieving targets for the promotion of specific drugs or products of certain pharmaceutical companies. The doctors are usually paid 1000 dollars just for advising a patient to buy certain drugs! As soon as the patient (who consider the doctor like a God) goes to get the drug, then they pay the money to the doctor!

They set up people who have nothing wrong with a false diagnosis, done electronically in labs, creating a need to take drugs for life, thus milking money for the pharmaceutical company, and ultimately leading to the patient's death. It is like the common saying, "The operation was successful but the patient died!". It was discovered that in the state of Minnesota, 100 of those beastly doctors received more than 100,000 dollars each for promoting the manufactured tests and diagnosis and suggesting certain drugs.

Other doctors were paid to give lectures to tell other doctors how important it is to have the drugs. Then these, in their turn, would also be paid generously. Some doctors take pay-off money from companies for going to various meetings to sit on the committees that have to test the drugs, acting as a mouthpiece for the company. The doctors who manage to persuade the audience to buy the drug are richly rewarded by the pharmaceutical company.

The phenomenon has reached a huge scale ... patients and relatives all over have started to scream about these unethical practices. In about a dozen interviews with doctors who have started to realize the consequences of such practices –not only of losing their license but also imprisonment – they said that the money they received had nothing to do with the health of the people they were "curing" !!! It was also established that the patients knew nothing at all of this money being paid to the doctors. Only a few patients knew what was going on and asked questions. For example, there are over forty drugs against cholesterol and the pharmaceutical companies try to persuade the doctors to prescribe their drug for a good payoff. Following up on revelations from Minnesota, a New York Times/CBS News poll last month found that 85 percent of respondents thought it "not acceptable" for doctors to be paid by drug companies to recommend their prescription drugs. Eighty-five percent also said such payments would influence the decisions that doctors made about patient care. ".

An email correspondent brought this article to my attention in August 2007.

I should have known by now, or expected something like this, but I didn't manage to sleep that night. The doctors were rewarded with 1000 dollars for each patient they put on the companies' drugs?

I remembered letters from Christos Riganas, from the Koridalos Prison where he was jailed for the possession and use of hashish, who fought against taking the AIDS pills. Every time he would return to jail, he would see that the inmates who took the drugs against AIDS were deteriorating rapidly. "Some new inmate had arrived and we were enthusiastically playing football in the prison yard. When I saw them again, next time I was in, they couldn't move because of the effects of the medication." Christos read newspapers, he sent the first letter to my attention at *"To Vima."* He wanted to be heard!

I got up at 5.00 am, to turn the computer on; I wanted to put a link to that medical corruption article on my web site, so that everybody could see it, and then go back to sleep more relaxed. But it was still not good enough. I added: "I stopped taking the drugs against AIDS on April 23rd 2007 and now feel perfectly fine," putting this in a rush on the front page of HIVwave.gr. It was as if I could hear the song by Akis Panou[33], "if this passes by, what could the rest do to me? This is the ocean and the rest is a drop...."

5. AIDS Experts have no answers

I remembered now again what happened when Nobel laureate Kary Mullis asked his research colleagues "Where are the papers" that show HIV causes AIDS; nobody could answer.

We obtained a similar result here in Greece. There was no answer to our formal request[34] to the Hellenic Center for Disease Prevention and Control (KEELPNO) for the proof of the concept that HIV cause AIDS. The question has also been asked in other countries; nobody can present any reliable evidence.

Lambros Papantoniou, the Greek Press correspondent, went to a special press briefing at the US State Department, with Ambassador Mark R. Dybul, Coordinator for the President's Emergency Plan for AIDS Relief (PEPFAR), on November 1st 2007.

He was the only reporter to ask questions at the briefing. And what did he ask??? An excerpt from the transcript: [35]

Question: [from Lambros Papantoniou, Greek correspondent of the

---

33 Akis Panou (1933-2000) Popular Greek music composer and singer of rebetiko songs
34 Posted in HIVwave.gr, in Greek only: Ζητάμε τις αποδείξεις.

35 U.S. Department of State, Ambassador Mark R. Dybul, Coordinator for the
    President's Emergency Plan for AIDS Relief (PEPFAR) On the Impact of Generic
    Antiretrovirals on HIV/AIDS Treatment Programs, Special Briefing, Office of the
    Spokesman, Washington, DC, November 1, 2007. Transcript at
    http://www.state.gov/r/pa/prs/ps/2007/nov/94522.htm

Greek daily newspaper, *Eleftheros Typos*, Athens]: Ambassador Dybul,'have you see the HIV virus in the laboratory?'

Ambassador Dybul: I've seen -- under a microscope, yes, I've seen photos -- electron micrographs of the virus. Yes.

Question: And where and when?

Ambassador Dybul: Oh, they're all over the place. They're published in virtually every journal. I have a picture of one in my office. [...]

Question: Ambassador Dybul, how do you allow U.S. doctors to prescribe this AIDS (inaudible) medication since they never saw the AIDS virus, as you say that is a part of (inaudible), but only pictures on the internet?

Ambassador Dybul: The reason we can do so is because the evidence is overwhelming that HIV exists. We have pictures. We have budding virus. We have the virus itself. We know what its inner workings look like through crystallography. There's a lot of things you can't see under a microscope that we -- a standard microscope -- you have to use high-powered technology. You need technological advances to see it, but we can see it. The data are overwhelming that it's transmissible, and the data are overwhelming that drugs that interfere with its replication lead to healthy patients. So from every standard of clinical medicine, it would be immoral to not use it.

The next day, I learned the details:

Maria, good morning! Just to inform you..... No other reporter asked any questions!!! And in the press hall, there were many representatives of the biggest pharmaceutical industries!!! Everybody in State Department is in alert, because millions of people around the world have watched a direct transmission of my dialogue.

With Gilles, we searched the Internet just for fun. *State Dept. official questioned by Dissident Reporter* was the title of one discussion topic in the AIDSMythExposed.com discussion forum. Here are some of their comments:

Just wondering where is the link for the brave Greek dissident reporter who courageously challenged the HIV=AIDS=DEATH dogma at a White House Press Conference...

"A friend of mine emailed a friend of his that lives in Athens, and from what I read in his email, the correspondent, Lambros Papantoniou, has never been controversial, he is much respected in Greece."

"The Greek respondent (reporter) was asking dissident questions nervously.. while Ambassodor Dybul swallowed his tongue, scouring for answers from his brain."

"Do you think the Greek reporter was the only reporter present? I'm sure the Ambassador was surprised at the dissident questions. He had all of the answers didn't he? [...] That was very interesting to watch and I think the reporter should be applauded."

On November 4th, we learned what Dr Maniotis thought of the exchange when Lambros phoned him. He said Mark Dybul lied when he said he had seen the virus, adding that nobody has ever seen the virus in AIDS patients.

A new message came from Lambros on 5th November :

It is a frenzy.....The opposite side is trying to overrun me. They call me the "hero" of the AIDS objectors on the website. They also asked the State Department to remove me from the accredited press correspondents group.

The icing on the cake: on November 11, Dr. George Pavlakis, a Greek-American professor in contact with Dr. Robert Gallo, advised Lambros to interview both Dr. Robert Gallo and Dr. John Moore, one of the most aggressive supporters of the AIDS orthodoxy. But I was to appear too now...

Maria, good morning! Early this morning I was phoned by Dr. Pavlakis after he had sent a message to my telephone-answering device. He told me that Robert Gallo and John Moore are going to give me a statement and an interview for World AIDS Day . I answered "with great pleasure". [But] Gallo demanded that I break off the communication with Maniotis and I cut it off, saying that this is impossible in any case. Then they required me not take interviews from the opposite side. I answered that it was my right to interview whomever and whenever I wanted and the reader then could judge what is right and what is wrong.

They're bothered because I communicate with you and because they have seen my writings on your web page. I gave the proper answer. Then, they say that you're lying when you write that you have not taken your medications since April, making other patients believe you and lose their lives! Simply, you must be taking the medication secretly. You could not have lived so long a time without medication!!! Good Lord!!!

In conclusion, he suggested that I should visit their laboratory where they will show me the virus with a special machine and their photographer will stand next to me, taking pictures that they will finally give me! I answered "with pleasure! I am ready". When that moment comes, I will also have with me a scientist of my choice, because very simply I don't trust them.

When I told Maniotis what had been said, he broke out into laughter.

A new message came on November 11th. This time Lambros told me that Dr. George Pavlakis had phoned him to give him Dr. John Moore's address so he could organize on Wednesday the first interview and be shown the virus.
And Lambros had an enjoyable answer, as always :

George, hello!
Thank you for Dr. John Moore's information. I will talk with him tomorrow so as not to disturb him on Sunday. I plan to meet him, and see the "virus", after you come back from your trip. Send me an email as soon as possible, and I will go to see the virus, as you said yesterday, taking the photograph with me as a souvenir. Have a nice trip
With friendly regards
Lambros

Next day, November 12, 2007, Lambros wrote to Dr. Moore:

My friend, Dr. George Pavlakis, has given to me your e-mail and your telephone number, in order to take from you a statement, and an interview, on the HIV/AIDS issue, due to the upcoming World AIDS Day, December 1st. At your convenience, let me know when you could be available. And how you would like to proceed, in writing or over the phone?
In expectation of your reply, I thank you very much!
Kind regards
Lambros Papantoniou

An immediate answer followed:

Dear Mr Papantoniou.
I'm unsure what you mean about an interview on the "HIV/AIDS" issue. Would you please clarify what is that you wish to discuss, specifically? I have also no wish to make a formal "statement" on any particular subject. If you have some specific questions to which you would like my answers, then please email them to me and I will decide whether to reply in writing or to conduct a telephone interview later this week.
Regards
John Moore

Lambros explained next day:

I have been advised by Dr. George Pavlakis to get in touch with you as an expert on "HIV/AIDS" issue. I don' t know the reasons. Please, get in touch with him, and then we could proceed accordingly (...)

New answer by Dr. Moore:

Dear Mr Papantoniou,
I am still giving your request some consideration, and will decide whether to agree in the next day or so. My concern about talking with you relates to the questions you recently asked Mark Dybul, the US

Global AIDS Coordinator, at a recent press conference in Washington. Those questions sounded very like they had been pressed onto you by Dr. Maniotis, the Greek-born scientist who does not believe that HIV either exists or is a public health threat, and who has stated on the Internet that he regularly talks to you about HIV/AIDS issues. I have no interest in contributing to any interview that further disseminates the kind of pseudoscientific nonsense that Dr. Maniotis believes in. Whether an interview with you on the real issues about HIV and its impact on global public health is possible is something that, as I say, I am still considering.

Regards
John Moore

The journalist's final answer:

Dear Dr. Moore,
Thank you for your recent communication concerning the possibility of an interview recommended by Dr. George Pavlakis. As you know this was not at my initiative and, therefore, I consider the matter closed and any discussion about personalities inappropriate.
Sincerely
Lambros Papantoniou

So, one of the most vocal accuser of the "dissidents" will not show him the virus, either alive or on a picture. He kept searching for reliable evidence of that virus. He was then contacted by the National Cancer Institute, where much AIDS research is carried out. On the 29th of November 2007, Mrs. Hardison, who works in the press office of the National Cancer Institution, got in touch to arrange an interview. Here is one relevant email:

Dear Mrs Hardison,
I would like to thank you for the conversation that we had few minutes ago, according to the e-mail that you had sent me. You wrote that my name has been given to you by a scientist because of my questions about the existence or not of the HIV virus. You also told me that the position of your work is a laboratory of the Ministry of Defense thus, you are able to answer nothing about HIV virus, but only general questions related to vaccines. I will respect it, there is no problem at all.

What does the National Cancer Institute has to do with the US Ministry of defense? Why would that render the employee unable to answer about the HIV virus. Are we talking about military secrets?

Anyway, later the same day, Lambros heard from the National Cancer Institute that his request was accepted, he could submit his questions in writing and they would answer him. He sent in 25 appropriate questions on the 1st of

December 2007, on vaccines and the relationship of HIV to AIDS. On December 5th, when he phoned the Institute, someone else answered and told him that their communications should be only written. On 19th of December, the reporter again tried in vain to learn when he could expect the answers. On 20 December they told him that the answers would be sent within 20 days; on 15 January 2008 he contacted the employee to whom he had first spoken on the phone who declared that she didn't know the reason for that delay; on 31 January 2008 somebody else answered the phone, saying that he didn't have any idea about the answers.

On the 1st of February 2008, two months after the initial application, the reporter found a message in his answer phone from an anonymous employee of the government, informing him that the National Cancer Institute was not going to answer his questions and he could address himself to another office.

So, apparently, the questions were not easy to answer in a way that would satisfy AIDS Public relations. They had no obligation to answer after all, and perhaps they did not want to touch the 'hot potato'.

But the results for us are the same: when asked fundamental AIDS questions, AIDS experts do not answer properly, nor do they have the answers. Is there anything substantial under the pseudo-scientific coat of the AIDS artificial construction?

6. Virus mania

To reinforce the popular fear of viruses, in parallel to the scandal of AIDS, the medical establishment seems to complement it with plenty of similar stories of apparently fatal diseases. In doing so, a new fashion in medical science has been launched, and the proof of this is in the book *"Virus Mania : How the Medical Industry Continually Invents Epidemics, Making Billion Dollar Profits at Our Expense"* (2007) by Torstein Engelbrecht, reporter, and Claus Köhhnlein, doctor.

Covering the viruses supposed to cause bird flu (H5N1), SARS, BSE, Hepatitis C, AIDS, polio, all of them of dubious identity and pathogenicity, the authors expose the reality behind the successive threats coming from viruses and draw the conclusion that the commercialization of medicine overpass the basic principles of science. And they show how the apparent lethal spread of the widely advertised germs has never been based on proper, ethical scientific criteria.

We cannot be fooled so easily any more. As shown in Greece by bloggers like Erinya, a teacher from Thessaloniki who powerfully draws parallels between religion and AIDS (http://erinya-hellenica.blogspot.com), and Maria Pateraki, a teacher in the island of Poros, who created the web blog *New World's Whispers* (http://newworldswhispers.blogspot.com) initially to help my endeavour. Here are her comments (in parentheses) on a related news article (translated from Greek):

Elefterotypia newspaper, Friday 24/8/07

The UN foresees a Worldwide Health Crisis of new Contagious Diseases.

"The preconditions are made for the appearance of new infectious diseases and the rapid spread of them by the modern communication means, WHO warns *(or rather I would say "terrifies")* highlighting the need for international cooperation to avert pandemics.

With millions of people wandering over the planet every year, diseases spread more rapidly than ever in history. Travelers can move around more easily and anywhere at any time, which makes it more likely for any disease to spread in some other parts of the world, and elsewhere in the globe within a few hours. *(Do you hear my words, curious traveler? Yes I do, you should say!)* In the last 5 years, WHO has registered worldwide over 1100 epidemics of dangerous diseases, like cholera, polio and bird flu *(where are the other 1097?)*. The fact is that today, man has access to more and more once distant and solitary areas that make dispersal more likely for more and more diseases. To be precise, we come face to face with a new epidemic every year. At the moment there are 39 Pathogenic Factors which were unknown a generation ago: among them are the viruses of AIDS *(here is another plural form, I can only imagine that they all belong to the HIV clan - What a clan, eh!)*, the hemorrhagic fever Ebola, the heavy respiratory syndrome SARS *(You should not too soon get ready for a trip to Africa or Asia. Stay home!)* As WHO pointed out *(Don't take it easy)* at the annual exhibition for worldwide health "it would be naive for anyone to think that it won't be another disease like AIDS, another Ebola or another SARS" *(since we have already made you guilty and fearful about having sex - shame on you, again, why not get you in now and scare you some more)*.

That is exactly the reason *(That only, believe me)* for which the organization has acted on reviewing the International Health Regulations and asks for the cooperation of all countries especially in informing WHO about the emergence of a new epidemic *(You can't play around with things like this!)*. Only through a global timely rally and the proper exchange of information will we be able to avoid the epidemics *(after having made you lose ten years of your life - in the common way - sweating and asking yourselves if you have caught anything!)*. All countries are also invited to share with each other and with WHO the viruses they have found so that they multiply attempts to develop vaccines against the viruses. *(Thank God, business is low!)*

We cannot complain though, we live in a world of great science fiction!

7. Mind control

The AIDS syndrome has appeared like a "political disease" from the beginning. But why should anyone introduce its "false reality" into our lives?

It certainly benefits a large number of people, for different reasons. One of these benefits was presented earlier in this chapter: it can be used to promote fear in the population under the guise of promoting safety.

Going a little back in history, the leaders of the mighty military-industrial complex was deeply affected by the antiwar movements of the sixties and seventies. They hated the Peace and Love movement; they were incensed by the slogan: "Make love, not war".

In 1984, under the puritan Reagan administration, the discovery of the so-called AIDS virus was proclaimed to the world during an International press conference, bypassing the regular scientific procedure. When the US Secretary for Health and Human Services, Margaret Heckler, announced that they had discovered a new dangerous retrovirus, almost nobody knew what this meant. Clever. And using spurious statistics, they were able to blame sex as a leading factor in the spread of this apparently new disease.

The 'AIDS' problem was presented as a complicated scientific issue so that nobody could doubt it. And we were told that soon science would find the solution, since science is powerful and dedicated to this fight.

For the average person, there was no urge to question the 'science,' since they were going to find the solution soon. And we have seen that the careers of scientists are threatened if they question 'AIDS science'. So most people remained captives of this belief, for twenty-five years so far (1984 – 2009).

The whole body of scientific literature is based on false assumptions, such as that HIV causes AIDS, or is sexually transmitted.

In the web page *"NomoreFakenews.com"*, John Rappoport (author of *AIDS Inc. Scandal of the Century*) presented an interview with Ellis Medavoy (pseudonym of a retired propaganda operative, who worked for various groups spreading lies about medical subjects such as AIDS and vaccines). Media mind control was his speciality.

'AN EXPLOSIVE INTERVIEW WITH ELLIS MEDAVOY: MIND CONTROL, MIND FREEDOM,' 2006-02-13[36]

Rappoport: First of all, as you've told me before, you were involved in spreading the lie that AIDS is basically one condition caused by HIV.

Answer: That's right. There was a group that knew this was all a lie, and they wanted "traction" in the press. They wanted the world to accept HIV as the cause of AIDS. They wanted plenty of stories planted in the media. So I accepted that assignment. I was, of course, not the only person doing this. This was a very big operation.

Rappoport: What was the purpose of the lie?
Answer: As with any major op, there were several purposes. I've explained most of it to you before. But, as you can see, the world has seen, in recent years, an explosion in PR and propaganda about so-called epidemics. West Nile, SARS, bird flu. Besides scaring people and getting them to accept any and all medical and political edicts, the idea is to bring nations of the world into a tighter connection – because when you have an international agency like the World Health Organization at the helm, telling governments what they have to do and can't do, the "community of nations" draws closer and closer together.
Rappoport: Basically, you're talking about the move toward globalism, the rule of the many by the few...

a. Public Relations, with a new category of AIDS experts

I had started to enjoy the agitation that I have caused in the last 2 years in our country, as if I had thrown a pebble into a lake and watched the water ripple and grow further and further apart. But I would always be disappointed at the end.

"A different point of view on AIDS. Devote a few minutes and read it. I think it is worth it. I read it and it was quite real, not false. Maybe we should wait for an expert to explain it all," the sympathetic bloggers would suggest to their visitors. They were losing the battle from the start, the way I had done for a long time by trusting the experts.

In the book *Trust us, we're Experts. How industry manipulates science and gambles with your future* (Penguin, New York 2002), the authors, Sheldon Rampton and John Stauber, offer an exposé on the manufacturing of "independent experts" by public-relations firms. The "father of Public Relations", Edward L. Bernays described that in his classic work *"Propaganda"* (1928). Since then, the media stage on which much of modern public life is conducted is used by two kind of experts – the spin doctors behind the scenes, and the visible experts that they select, cultivate, and promote for public consumption.

What these experts express becomes our reality, courtesy of the media. Very few "independent experts," or journalists, find out or expose possible conflicts of interest. In that way, the Public Relations companies and the powerful elite that hire them may deceive courts, legislators, media and the public worldwide.

The implementation of the lie about AIDS becomes all the more complicated, incomprehensible for the many, a privilege for the few, which is the desired effect for the experts of Public Relations.

An image of the dead end now reached in this field was given by the professor of African History at the University of California Dr. Charles Geshekter, describing the situation in Africa:

Doctors find out that they lack basic pharmaceutical stuff, have few personnel, that their budget has been wiped out the last fifteen-twenty years, but that there is plenty of money to distribute printed matter regarding AIDS, condoms, and – the most harmful in my opinion – the so-called pharmaceutical treatment for AIDS.

b. Censorship. The "invisible" books of the dissidents

Suddenly I felt a strong impulse to read all the "prohibited" books in our house, those questioning the official version of 'AIDS'. I started devouring them, they seemed to never stop revealing the plain truth, even if they overlapped each other. We already had more than a dozen of them, and new ones were coming up almost every season.

Here are a few of the unknown aspects of the 'AIDS' construction:

More AIDS "patients" have to be created to give the impression of a growing epidemic. Easy: the AIDS definition changed six times since 1982. Robert Root–Bernstein in his book (*Rethinking AIDS. The tragic cost of premature consensus*, 1993, p. 67) explains the way the 'epidemic' appeared to be growing:

> Much of our public health policy rests upon calculations of how fast AIDS is growing and into what groups it seems to be spreading. Each time the definition of AIDS changes, all of these calculations change as well. Previously excluded people suddenly qualify as AIDS patients. Diagnoses sky-rocket. The 1985 definition change resulted in 2000 additional cases a year in U.S. The 1987 revision resulted in about a 30 percent increase in diagnoses, or some 10,000 new cases in 1988 and some 15,000 additional cases during 1991. The proposed 1992 definition may double the number of diagnoses overnight.

Nobody reacted, ever? Even when there were investigations about scientific misconduct, they were derailed

As Janine Roberts showed in her book *Fear of the Invisible* [37], "there have been astonishingly five major investigations between 1990 and 1995 into possible fraud in Gallo's HIV research, several of which overlapped each other". The clearest evidence of criminal fraud was unearthed by the Dingell Inquiry in 1993 and "was immediately presented to the State Attorney General in January 1994 in the expectation that a criminal prosecution would now be ordered, but he ruled it was 'out of time'. Too long had elapsed under the Stature of Limitations since the fraud was carried out. Gallo thus may have escaped prosecution on a technicality."

Dingell was a Democratic Congressman, and when the Republican Party took control of the House of Representatives at the end of 1994, he lost his

---

37 Janine Roberts, *Fear of the Invisible*, Impact Investigative Media Productions, 2008, pp. 108, 113, 115

chairmanship of the investigating sub-committee, and the Republicans promptly killed the investigation of the Reagan-endorsed Robert Gallo.

The findings of all these high level investigations of the 1990s were thus swiftly and shockingly buried. Few AIDS scientists now know that these seminal AIDS papers were thoroughly discredited by scientists belonging to the most eminent of scientific bodies. This is an extraordinary state of affairs. It is totally amazing, almost unbelievable. It is as if these highly prestigious top-level investigations never existed - yet they only completed their work in 1995.

In 1996, *Impure Science* (University of California Press) by Steven Epstein, professor of Sociology at the University of California in San Diego, suggested that "If, as some have sought to argue, the "purity" of science is guaranteed by its insulation from external pressures, then AIDS research is a clear-cut case of impure science." (p.8)

As for the 'scientific consensus' which keeps AIDS alive, Michel Crichton said: "The greatest scientists in history are great precisely because they broke with the consensus ... There is no such thing as consensus science. If it's consensus, it isn't science. If it's science, it isn't consensus. Period."

It is relatively easy to create a consensus artificially, as is described by Laurence E. Badgley, M.D. in the foreword of Jon Rappoport's book. *AIDS Inc. Scandal of the century* (1998):

Truth is usually simple. Yet the AIDS virus theory has entered a realm of scientific obfuscation. Our addiction to animal research provides us with faulty information about AIDS and drugs intended for humans who differ physiologically from other species. In the entire world today there are only approximately 200 scientists who understand the inner-circle language and symbols of esoteric virology. From sterile and isolated sancta, these 'Priests of Virology' have handed down their own interpretation of the 'Higher Knowledge' of Nature. These few Priests have informed the millions of doctors of the world as to 'how things are' with this disease called AIDS.

In other words, only about 200 scientists needed to be discouraged from speaking out. The rest of the scientists and the medical community would not understand they were being fooled, and would follow the proclamations of the virology experts.

Even more so for the doctors. They depend on and defer to authority. That's how they work ! (Robert Root- Bernstein " *Rethinking AIDS*"[38]. They are keen

---

38 Robert Root-Bernstein, Rethinking AIDS: *The Tragic Cost of Premature Consensus*, Free Press, 1993, 512 pages. p. 353-354.
   Dr. Robert Root-Bernstein, who held a MacArthur Prize fellowship from 1981 to 1986, is associate professor of physiology at Michigan State University.

to quote authority:

> Recent studies by Dr. Thomas Chalmers of Harvard University and Marlys and Charles Witte and Ann Kirwan of the University of Arizona, among others, have demonstrated that physicians are perhaps the most authority oriented of all professionals. They are evaluated in medical school not on the basis of their critical thinking skills, their creativity, or their independence, but their ability to learn quicky, to memorize well, to act prudently, and to be able to quote authority extensively. They want and are paid for having answers, not questions

We think that the DNA of the HIV virus has been identified. Really? Despite the fact that Gallo himself has admitted, at a 1994 meeting sponsored by the US National Institute of Drug Abuse, "We have never found HIV DNA in T-Cells"[39], the researchers started working on its DNA decryption. From the book by Jean Claude Roussez *SIDA, Supercherie scientifique et Arnaque humanitaire* (p.33), here is the outcome:

> Normally all the DNA duplicates should correspond with each other, since they come from the same virus. But not one was the same as the others! After discovering this, surely the inventors of the virus should have questioned their initial assumptions? But, we would be naive to expect something like that. It seemed better for them to suggest a virus with a thousand faces, a wildly mutating virus. Soon we had at least a hundred variations of it. Today they are countless.

Why did we endorse so easily this theory that viruses can wildly mutate themselves and yet be the same virus?

Celia Farber, in the book *Serious Adverse Events. An Uncensored history of AIDS* (Melville House Publishing, 2006), states that:

> Winston Churchill famously said: "The empires of the future are the empires of the mind". This was during his spell of enthusiasm for the implementation of a lingua franca used by the Allies called Basic English, a language of only 850 words. George Orwell, during his years at the BBC, was himself interested in Basic, and scholars say it formed the basis of the totalitarian language "Newspeak" in 1984.
>
> Since April 23, 1984, an empire of the mind has been expanding around our world. It is a simple, terrifying idea, and each mind in which it implants becomes incorporated, as territory, into the empire. It was not really an idea but more of a dictum. Colossally powerful, the dictum was that there was a single sexually transmissible virus that would bring imminent death upon millions of Americans.

---

39 *The fear of the Invisible*, op.cit. p. 132

Meanwhile, that AIDS dictum is constantly being contradicted by reality, but has remained powerful, because most people do not really understand what it is all about.

Gilles made an improvised survey in his class of Modern Greek for foreigners that he was attending at the University of Athens. He handed out a questionnaire to his classmates with two questions only: Do you know anyone who is HIV-positive? How many men/ women? The 16 foreigners, from all around the world (Ukraine, Russia, Spain, Germany, Romania, Turkey and elsewhere), answered No, None, None. One student from Congo, who did not understand the question properly, answered "5%." Conclusion: Where is the big AIDS epidemic?

However, wherever they are, the HIV-positive persons are invisible to society. Unless they are being used like moving advertisements for 'AIDS prevention' and medication, just like Magic Johnson who tours the world sponsored by the pharmaceutical industry.

"Like the prisoners at Auschwitz who were known only by numbers, that's what we are like", Helen, an HIV-positive friend from Crete told me the other day. I remembered the unspeakable fear I had felt when I saw my file the very first day – the doctors proudly explained to me that I had become anonymous, Mpap, together with a number. All that I was, that I had achieved, that the others were waiting from me, had become a cypher, a monogram, I did not exist in the eyes of society.

The second surprise came at the hospital, when I entered my doctor's secondary office to ask a question, and noticed the shelves on the wall. They contained files with names written on them. Ah, there are our proper files, I thought, as I recognized some names. Why couldn't I find my name though? I looked again, in vain. "Who are they?" I asked at the end. "They are the ones who died", the doctor answered. After death we would take back our identity. What about our lost dignity?

So here's what happens with that new category of captives: instead of being pushed into gas chambers, they are poisoned slowly and silently. They are to be openly shown only if it is to say, "We now live well with the new AIDS medication"...

Chapter 6

Alternative realities: How I regained control of my health

1. Future Mom

It was September, five months after stopping AIDS medication, and I was working out at the gym and strongly suspecting that I was pregnant. Why not? I had recently had many nights of generous lovemaking with Gilles, since we had both agreed that I was ready for the big step. I thought as soon I decided on it then it would happen. I had become pregnant by accident when I was 20 and had to terminate. Why wouldn't it happen now when I wanted it? Moreover, even while sick with 'AIDS', my gynecological tests were always good.

I was mumbling a song along with that wishful thinking while on the stationary bicycle, when one of my liveliest friends, Irene Constantinou, the gym teacher, came up to me and asked: "Getting ready for the baby?" "I don't know. I feel fine but I must build the strength to take this pregnancy. What do you think? How will I do?" Irene knew I was an AIDS patient. "Are you joking? You will be beating us all up in no time at all". Of course she was not aware about my past history of medication damage, but I had almost forgotten it myself.

I decided to make my first visit to the gynecologist that a co-worker, Joanna Soufleri, who was my age and also pregnant with her first child, had recommended. "You must know more about AIDS than I do" were the first words out of the doctor's mouth. See, another kind doctor. I had gone to him in advance and put the case like that: "I want to have a baby, I am HIV positive. If I get pregnant, will you take me on?" He didn't seem disturbed at all. "You will have to speak with your AIDS doctor first. Have you heard of the protocol of HIV? You will have to follow that," he said simply. I replied: "I've come to you to avoid the AIDS doctors, as suggested by Dr. Maniotis, a specialist, a great American researcher, a teacher in one of the largest medical schools in Chicago, in the USA. We were constantly in touch via the Internet and he said I have nothing to worry about. Let us suppose I wasn't HIV positive. Let us pretend that I am pregnant and came to you on my own, what happens then?" "I can take you on just like any other woman who comes to me. When the time comes for you to give birth, you will have to go to maternity hospital. There it is obligatory to have tests of antibodies for HIV and if you are found HIV-positive, then you'll be called on by a council of specialists to decide what AIDS medicine will be given you the last 3 months of your pregnancy so that your baby is born healthy.

"Medicine?" I growled " Can we skip protocol? I have been waiting for months to detox myself from the AIDS drugs and now you tell me that by having a baby I have to take them again?" He told me: "It is not up to me at the point. To have the baby you have to go to the maternity hospital. There, they are obliged to go by protocol. It is law, I am telling you. We cannot go against the laws." Surely, how can this kind of law be? It is against human rights, only the person involved should have the right to accept or decline any tests or therapy. Besides, there is also the natural law which prohibits criminality. Giving toxic medication to pregnant women and their child should be considered criminal. How can we now bypass that mistaken medical law? "Until the time for me to go to the hospital, will you keep an eye on me?" "If you get pregnant naturally, no problem. Will do whatever I should usually do. I could not have known you are HIV-positive. But where will you have the baby? "I will ask for a midwife, just like the old times. Do not worry, Christine Maggiore did the same in Los Angeles."

"I am sorry, but I am going to be the devil's advocate " the doctor said now. "If your child, and I say if, because we have to view all possibilities – if he turns out to be seropositive in a few years, what will you say to him?" "I will explain to him about the AIDS deception, I will tell what happened to its mother and he will understand." I am writing this calmly now but I started losing my temper in front of the doctor. I kept on hearing repeatedly everyone, nice people, educated, trying to be polite but turned out to be dangerously deceived.

"Are the objections that you refer to in Pubmed?" He asked me troubled. I knew the answer. It was a SOS question as we used to say at school during examinations. Somebody else had already asked me on the website a similar question. Actually he had found out that all my reports are wrong since they were not included in Pubmed. What an argument! What is this Pubmed?

I had asked Gilles. It used to be the golden bible of the doctors, but it had been overpassed in our time. I had crushed that reader with some vivid examples, but I didn't need to say much now. "Pubmed has been denounced for being choosy of what medical articles it publishes," I said very sure of myself. "What are you talking about? I've an article published in there" he reacted. "Well, surely your article did not question the dominant dogma " I felt like I was little by little losing an ally. And I was then in a hurry to say goodbye. "Will try to get pregnant naturally. If it happens, I will be coming back to you". We uncomfortably said goodbye to each other. I would leave him some time to think about it.

A few days later, during an appointment with my homeopath. I told him about difficulties that popped up and the possibility that they would have to give me the drugs during the last 3 months of the pregnancy, even if I managed it alone. He tried to cheer me up a bit by saying: "If you rush in to have a baby, you won't have the time to take the last three months drugs, so what is the problem?" But they might give, my newborn baby the drugs or to me while I am asleep, they are fanatical about that. "They will not know that you are seropositive, you will surprise them". What an anxiety before giving birth to your child! "Maybe it is better not to go at all and find a midwife if needed?" "We will find whatever you want." "I will see you in 2 months" I said happily now.

"What kind of programming is this?" "In November my detoxification period expires." "How do you know so precisely? Do you have an appointment with Mother Nature? "That is how long my American doctor told me to wait until..." Did he give you a general plan, aren't you going to check your watch now? Stress doesn't help. And do you think as soon as you decide to have a baby it will happen? Have you decided on a boy or girl?" "I have already thought of a name." "If you feel O.K why not start trying now....?"

But we had already started. I left flying high. This homeopath was more like a psychologist, he put me in a good mood. The basic thing was for me to get pregnant naturally. So many women for centuries have done it this way. I liked the idea of following that time honored tradition.

Everything looked like I was already pregnant. I was sleepy all the time, eating continuously and looked radiant. Then I had the idea to do a home pregnancy test a few days before the first signs would show. There were some new tests on the market that showed the results 4 days before the next menstruation. I went to the pharmacy and bought a kit. I did it. I had to wait 3 minutes for it to show 2 lines. However, it could show it in 1 minute. It showed it in half a minute. Gilles...!!! I shouted. I knew it. We both knew it . We were ready for this. "You're wonderful" my beloved one said to me. He went out for a while and came back with a bunch of blue-mauve-turquoise hydrangeas and a bottle of wine. We were expecting my mother to come over and celebrate. In addition, the phone went wild. Soon, all of my friends had heard about it, well nearly all of them. "Shouldn't we confirm it first?" "No, it is definite" we both had decided. Of course, there would be tests to be taken the next day. And the first and main test: was negative. They said the chemical test was wrong. And I was so sure of the things I was feeling. For two whole days. They called it self-suggestion, I think. And why did I rush to announce it to everyone? "Impatience is a flaw" my brother used to tell me. I feared I would be told this again, but he didn't say. Who would dare tell me after 12 years of patience and another 6 months of detoxification?

Everyone was trying to comfort me in another way. "It is not so easy to conceive a baby from the first month. The possibilities are 25% for all normal couples", the second gynecologist that I visited also said, "other women try for years". Even so, I rejoined the majority of the female population, I was not an exception any more. I was going to the doctor's waiting room and calming down. Just being there was a conquest for me, and I felt better with that second doctor. It looks like he wanted to take me on with more good humor. "What else can we do?" He would say and try to find new ideas. We would have to start the traditional way by waiting month after month and then if nothing happened we would go on another method. Saying the last words, he seemed to carry a culpable smile. As for himself, he was covered by the medical secrecy. But any other method was actually out of question if we wanted to avoid unfortunate surprises from the AIDS establishment.

We would start a new trick: "We are going to see when your next ovulation is, it would be better for you, and Gilles not have sexual contact 2 or 3 days earlier. It is the traditional way to make conception more likely, because the sperm is more concentrated" the doctor advised. He would be from now on a new cordial ally, but Gilles wasn't very happy about this last suggestion and found on the Internet that same night an article saying the opposite "Daily sex can help repair sperm, says fertility doctor." I could not resist laughing. "You went and found the opposite by some other guy on the Internet?" "Not at all. It is a new development in research that has been printed in two big newspapers" I looked at the articles again, the first from The Times 16th October 2007 and the 2nd from Guardian 16th October 2007. It was the 21st October then .He left me astonished again. "Why should we believe that now?" I hesitantly asked. I wanted to follow the doctor's advice, he was the only doctor I would need anymore. However, my loved one had a different hunch and that was enough for me. He started singing the song by Leonard Cohen, a promise he had given to me before coming to Athens: "If you want a boxer, I will step into the ring for you…. And if you want a doctor, I will examine every inch of you…."

Later on, he sent me an e-mail from the next room.

"Dear Maria
It seems that an important aspect of the AIDS deception has been forgotten in your "Adios AIDS" book. [40]
The fear of love instilled by the sexual AIDS myth had a tremendous impact on our society. By 1987, it had killed the sexual revolution. Effectively dismissed the Peace and Love movement.
- In the USA, promoting sexual abstinence is now the preferred strategy (officially) to prevent 'HIV' infection.
- With the 'HIV' pretense, some people are sent to jail after consensual sex.   Never mind the health benefits of love, and sex.

It could be important for your readers to get a short summary of those benefits, because "Today's public discourse about sexuality is almost exclusively about risks and dangers. Public discourse about the physiological and psychosocial health benefits of sexual expression has been almost entirely absent" as mentioned in the introduction of a study presented during the 1st World Congress for Sexual Health, in April 2007 (It was actually published by Planned Parenthood in 2003)[41]:

In 1994, the 14th World Congress of Sexology adopted the Declaration of Sexual Rights. This document of "fundamental and

---

[40] As mentioned in my short PeaceandLove.ca 'AIDS' biography (http://www.peaceandlove.ca/gstpintro.htm)

[41] The Health Benefits of Sexual Expression Published in Cooperation with the Society for the Scientific Study of Sexuality

universal human rights" included the right to sexual pleasure. This international gathering of sexuality scientists declared, "Sexual pleasure, including autoeroticism, is a source of physical, psychological, intellectual and spiritual well-being" (WAS, 1994).

Despite this scientific view, the belief that sex has a negative effect upon the individual has been more common in many historical and most contemporary cultures. In fact, Western civilization has a millennia-long tradition of sex-negative attitudes and biases. In the United States, this heritage was relieved briefly by the "joy-of-sex" revolution of the '60s and '70s, but alarmist sexual viewpoints retrenched and solidified with the advent of the HIV pandemic. Today's public discourse about sexuality is almost exclusively about risks and dangers: abuse, addiction, dysfunction, infection, pedophilia, teen pregnancy, and the struggle of sexual minorities for their civil rights. Public discourse about the physiological and psychosocial health benefits of sexual expression has been almost entirely absent (Davey Smith et al., 1997; Reiss, 1990).

However, pioneering researchers have demonstrated many of the various health benefits of sexual expression, including its positive physical, intellectual, emotional, and social dimensions (Ogden, 2001). [...] I can provide more details if you wish.

Love, love, love

Gilles

Soon afterward, ignorant of the lattest developments, a reporter asked to do an interview, not with me, but with Gilles. But he addressed me first: "If you agree to let your partner talk..." as if I had Aladdin's lamp. Well, it wasn't completely a lie. A lot of people wanted to learn about him but referred to me. I was so privileged after all! He inspired the whole world, people that had never met him. Another e-mail had arrived early on, just after my second book came out on March 29th 2007, and it said:

First of all my wife and I want to give a big 'well done' to your husband. Even though many people are prejudiced against those who are HIV positive (of course he was already educated), he still came from America and you had good news. I am 35 years old and my wife is 30, just so we know each other a bit. So, tell him that he is a "pallikari"!!! (a word he may not understand because of his lineage, but tell him we use it in Greece for the daring). I understand the state of fear in all its glory. I will remind you here of the word Vakoufika. You may not know it either but it describes the things that belong to the church and that no one is to touch, for the fear of God's wrath.

P.S I will send you the bill for the time I was absent from my job, doing a little research (I am joking).

In the meantime, our second attempt at pregnancy failed and we were trying for a third fertility period, when "X" turned up and asked me how I was doing since I stopped the pills? Without a second thought, I sent him by e-mail the latest version of the book I had started writing, the one you are reading now. I did this quite often; straight after this question, I would send the beginnings of the book to anyone who honestly wanted to know how I was. But this time "X" reprehended me "Do not ever do anything like that again" he said. "We do not ever show the book we are writing before publishing it."

I was quite put out, "Why, who could impersonate me?" I asked arrogantly. He admitted that it was hard to steal my glory and immediately changed his mood. He said that it was good that he had got to know me better, since I was uncovering so much about myself. That way he could help me the more. There was no reason for me to continue going to the homeopath, as he depended on the existence of symptoms to adjust and remove the cause of the pathology. But maybe it would be better to wait a little bit longer to go ahead with a pregnancy. "There's no way that I am going to wait any longer" I announced on the telephone call that followed straight after. "You have waited so many years, don't rush into something hasty. You have to be strong to go through with it." He added in a calm voice before we got off the phone; 'I would think about it for hours.'

One trip to his lab would give me enough information, but meanwhile he sent me an article that described my situation: "what is the natural reaction of the body to chemical medicine? The body reacts to the "chemical attack" of the drug, creating symptoms. As long as the first side effects of the drug last, it means that the body is fighting against its efficacy. This reaction however cannot go on forever. First of all, if it carries on producing symptoms of that kind, it could do permanent damage and secondly, because the human body doesn't have cellular memory, it is not regulated to cope with chemical reactions of this kind. The founder of homeopathic medicine, Samuel Hahnemann, in his inspired work "Organon of Medicine" (1842, 6th edition) wrote: "Only against natural diseases can God help with homeopathy [...] There is not and can't be a human cure for the recovery of the many abnormalities that so often are caused by allopathic malpractice."

The founder also stated, commenting on the abuse of chemical medicine in his time that still continues today: "Because of these cures, the vital force on the one hand weakens and on the other hand, if it doesn't succumb, it gets little by little disordered in a peculiar way according every different use of medicine. To keep up with life despite the hostile attacks, the vital force has to distort the body and deprive it of, or to modify, or to increase, some of its natural reactions."

"'X'" could take me on for as long as he needed, as long as I was punctual for my visits. The first visit was arranged. Of course, I went with Gilles and it was an unbelievable experience. First, he placed my fingertips and toes on a Kirlian machine[42] that recorded energy emissions on a photographic print. Then he

---

42 Kirlian Machine: It records the energy emissions of the body on a photographic print. Acupuncture points coincide with the energy patterns emanating from the subject,

inspected these photos thoroughly. Gilles wanted to check the thoroughness of the information that he was giving us so he did the same tests straight after me.

After analyzing the energetic prints, '"X"' started his treatment on the affected acupuncture points with a small pressurized electrical stimulation that let out all the pressure that had been jammed up all these years. The body parts that have not been too much affected by their pathology (regardless of the cause of it) still have a certain " fluidity" or "mobility" in them, he explained. They react strongly straight away. Moreover, only if the points of acupuncture have been chosen rightly, that is causatively and not symptomatically, will the body react in the right direction.

My body reacted strongly, that was a good sign. He concluded that I must have had a strong constitution and have taken good care of myself to appear so well after all of the so-called 'AIDS' diseases. The general picture for me was "above satisfactory".

That did not mean the absence of a deeper turmoil, or even damage. He said "a forest look fine when seen from a distance; closer, you see the broken branches, dry leaves, thinned outgrowth". He carried on: "Your pictures are very good in many ways. Rarely do we see people with such an absence of energetic pathological phenomena in those pictures. It is important though to understand that, up to a point, it is as important to fight against mental or biological shocks that have been formed during childhood as it is to fight against toxic medicine. I do not mean to emphasize or accuse one or the other, less or more so. But we say that each person is his own case. He is unique.

We come from the whole of our history, not just from one or another diagnostic method but from all of it together. If we can't conceive of and can't handle this as a whole, then the patient can't be helped. The key to unlocking his pathology may lay exactly at the point we haven't checked. That is why all diagnostic methods are respected from any medical system, as long as they are not harmful – some of them (thank god not many) are harmful indeed. That's how I was trained to think. Only thus can a curing system be called a "holistic." It can't otherwise, for example, find the right points for acupuncture or the right homeopathic medicine or even more the right surgery. This is because no method can find out everything, and because most of them, if not all, cannot act everywhere, not locally or quality or quantity wise".

Afterwards he put a crystal on my forehead and left me lying there for 5 minutes. "It might seem witchcraft but it does work, you will know". Little by little, something started to swell and gradually rise up towards my throat as though to strangle me. I turned towards him, and thankfully he was still there, right by me, watching, observing. He asked me what exactly was I feeling and if I could take it a little longer so he would not have to remove the crystal. I told him that I could and he left it on a little while longer, until he lifted it off gently from my forehead and left me nearly hypnotized and tranquil, adding sparingly on purpose, as he later told me. "That is just a sample of what's inside of you." He added slowly "and thank goodness you had a small outburst for it helped to

---

disturbances in the electromagnetic field can be diagnosed and treated.

unblock your inner chest". There followed a conversation with myself and Gilles, and stern advice to go to sleep. That night I slept so deeply it was as if I did not exist. "Only that kind of sleep rejuvenates the body" he had said "and we want you to regain that forever."

Oh, how I really wanted that! But stress wouldn't let me. I hoped for a time with no stress: "After December 1st the pressure that I am feeling now may release, and I will relax" I told him. "You won't be able to relax, because you have pressure gathered from all those years" my new therapist answered and then added: "Chronic use of repressive chemical drugs , that is the drugs that repress the symptoms and not the causative predisposition of the organism, drive the disease deeper to the more vital systems of the human body, including the psychic and intellectual, just the way homeopathy teaches us"

He would now target this, or whatever else were needed in my case. His method was unheard-of. It wasn't the usual acupuncture, the one with needles or electrical currents. Nor was it homeopathy, psychotherapy, going back hypnosis, or anything else that is well known. It was a different system, as he explained. They were alternative methods that anyone can study during or after university that deal with problems the medical system has given up on. He told me of other curing methods, such as osteopathy, biophysical and psychiatric orgone therapy, the most recent revolutionary "German New Medicine (GNM) by Dr Hamer, etc., and said each one had their own advantages. We should mix them up. They are all different things.

The homeopathy that I had started with had produced results, but it could not help much more. He would take me on. We started with one treatment that day and we would carry on with other therapies at future sessions which would be free of charge for me.

Another visionary had come my way. And he was good-looking again. Smart, gentle, well-educated. "Why is it so dangerous for you if somebody finds out that you are helping me?" I asked. " No, it is not dangerous, but I will explain to you later, " he said.

Later on he did tell me. I was surprised when he explained that he didn't take on other patients for treatment but that his activities were generally in research, papers and elsewhere. He told me his specific method, even though very efficient, is also vulnerable to attacks and criticism because of its nature (i.e. the use of crystals), and the whole idea of it might produce reactions against those working with alternative therapies in general. "They will say things like…. look what may happen to the ignorant ones when in desperation or deception they get away from the trail of medical method, and end up visiting and letting being used by speculators who cash in on human pain and hope, selling them frauds with crystals, needles and any other nonsense". That was enough reason for him to take me on free of charge for however long needed be. By exception.

It was unambiguous, I didn't insist at that point, I had my mind elsewhere. He told me, amongst other things, that my body was run-down from the afflictions I had suffered and because of my age – but we should not give up hope. He assured me that it wasn't impossible for me to conceive a baby, but that it would be difficult to hold on to it. Maybe I was in an intermediate phase, where the balance could not decide which way to sway, and his therapies would work to make it point in the right direction. He advised me to carry on with homeopathy for at least two weeks after my last visit to him. I pointed out that Hahnemann had said in the article he sent me that "There is not and can't be a human therapeutic art for the rehabilitation of the millions abnormalities that are caused by allopathic clumsiness.'

His answer was somehow disarming: "Is it enough to tell you that most people who find homeopathy a satisfactory solution today, have previously gone through what Hahnemann calls "allopathic clumsiness? "
And more into the specifics:

> "Homeopathy, depending on the stage at which it is applied, may save the organism from the damage done by chemical drugs, but only up to a point. Unfortunately, it cannot always completely repair the damage, even if applied from the start, because some chemical drugs, mostly vaccines, contain essences that take hold on the organism and are never eliminated – for example, the neurotoxic metals aluminium and mercury that are in various vaccines and tooth fillings. Homeopathy may reverse the situation if the chemical medicine exposure is current. A well known rule of homeopathy says that if an "A" illness is not rightly treated, then it is oppressed - that is, it apparently goes deeper as the outward symptoms go away (these symptoms being no more than the signs of effort by the organism to discard the illness) - and substantially it seeps deeper into more vital areas of the organism, to reappear there in a new, much more severe, and different form as "B" illness. Homeopathy treatment then may cure the "B" illness only to have the "A" illness reappear. It will be cured also if it isn't already too late – that is, if permanent organic damage has not been caused (in case of an organic disease) or if the health level has not dropped down to its bottom, where homeopathy alone cannot really help. Then other methods will be needed until the organism recuperates and returns to the higher health levels, from which it may be helped to disengaged from the original illness with the help of homeopathy, whenever possible.
>
> Sure, the best possible solution would be to start with homeopathy, so that the patient wouldn't need to pass through this Golgotha. Unfortunately many of the people who appeal to it are those who earlier didn't know about it, or didn't believe that it could help; because they heard others saying that their disease is "not curable," or did not trust it due to the way it is attacked and slanderered by those who feel it it may harm their interests."

All the same, I could not see any other solution. But it was impossible to continue the therapies with "X" as long as the research into my past was continuing. I felt it was more important for my new appearance in the world to finish that book, putting everything in order, than anything else. I also wished to get pregnant soon, the way it would happen in the old good days. But where would this blessed event take place, if it would ever come true? My good gynaecologist reassured me to help me calm down.

I now sent the news to my brother. He had often been valuable at the critical points of this route. Although he didn't live far away, he sent me this contribution by email:

> "Maria, I send you a few links for home childbirth. A daring, but also inexpensive alternative, that has found several supporters abroad"

An ultimate solution at my age...

2. The AZT baby conundrum

I believed until recently that AZT was not given to babies here in Greece or in other countries, except maybe in Africa. I believed this until we received the visit of a 'HIV-positive' healthy pregnant mother who had been told to start taking two anti-retroviral pills, Kaletra (2 protease inhibitors) and Combivir (AZT + 3TC), in the fifth month of her pregnancy because she was found positive with one of the unreliable 'HIV' tests during her regular prenatal checkup. She had thrown the Kaletra and Combivir into the trunk of her car and didn't know what to do with them. They should be spoilt by now due to the heat. But she didn't want to have them anyway.

The gynaecologist "could not undertake her case any longer" and the AIDS doctor simply gave her the toxic pills for the last three months of pregnancy and told her that AIDS doctors would be present during her caesarean delivery in order to take the baby immediately afterwards to the "Agia Sofia" children's hospital. There it would be given Retrovir syrup (AZT) for 40 days.

So, AZT really is given to babies here in Greece; It is used at the "Agia Sofia" hospital in downtown Athens.

"For me it was the reason I started my Internet activities in 1996", Gilles said , "when we started giving it to pregnant mothers in Canada. I consider it a crime. I kept quiet about the lack of evidence for sexual transmission since 1984, because it only affected my own sexual life. Besides, those people who took the 'AIDS' pills had a choice. However, babies and pregnant women do not have that choice, they are forced to poison their children (in Canada and USA). In Greece, the babies are actually taken away from their mothers for 40 days, so that 'AIDS' doctors can enforce their (mis-)treatment. In the USA those babies are then given an antibiotic (Bactrim) "to prevent future infections" and an AZT syrup called Retrovir even if the baby does not test 'HIV' positive. They send the police to mothers who refuse to give their baby AZT, and threaten to take permanent custody of the child. We are all responsible for letting that happen, with our taxes. It no longer concerns only people in the AIDS risk groups".

The 'AIDS' doctors probably never looked at the scientific studies on the toxicity of AZT. Nor had they seen the BBC documentary *"Guinea Pig Kids"*, by the investigative journalist Liam Scheff, and the articles in the press that led to it:

> Sean was 13. He weighed 50 pounds and was about four feet tall. An AZT baby. Stunted, his cells damaged from the inside out. I approached one of the children in a wheelchair, a boy about 12. There was something strange in his face—his head was oddly shaped. It was a bit squashed, with the eyes spaced widely. His limbs and torso were slightly warped, shortened and weak-looking. This is what happens to AZT babies.
> From _Orphans on Trial,_ New York Press, July 13, 2004

Maybe not every baby is so badly affected, but who wants to take that risk? Would the AIDS doctors perform that "therapy" on their own children? They probably do not think at all, otherwise I could not explain why with our new friend they insisted on knowing the exact date and place of the birth, so that they be sure to be there.

I was really shaken by that visit, it almost sent me back to 1995, making me desperate. What would my friend do next day when the AIDS doctors expected her? I remembered Dr. K.told us on our last visit that pills would only be given to me during the last three months of pregnancy, not to the baby – he said they seemed to have stopped doing the latter. So I suggested to her that she should tell her AIDS doctor that she now planned to continue her therapy with another AIDS doctor who did not prescribe medication for the baby, so that the first one would leave her alone and the second one would not know about this. It seemed to me like a good way of escaping – but my anxieties would not go away.

Then, another thing came to my mind. In his latest book _"Are you positive?"_ Stephen Davis had a brilliant idea for when communications with the AIDS doctors failed. [43] His solution summarized was:

> If you were diagnosed HIV-Positive, is there anything you can do? The answer is a resounding YES! [...] Read through the following list of things that would constitute lack of informed consent, and if you find one or more that are true in your own case, keep reading when you're finished with the list:
>
> 1) I was not informed that there were risks associated with merely taking an HIV test (the risk of mistakenly destroying your life), as stated by the Los Angeles County Department of Public Health on their web site
>
> 2) I was not informed that the FDA has never approved any test for the diagnosis of HIV infection.
>
> 3) I was not informed that the so-called HIV tests are not a test for HIV but for HIV antibodies
>
> 4) I was not informed that there is no recognized standard for establishing the presence or absence of antibodies to HIV-1 and HIV-2

---

[43] See pages 363-4.

in human blood, as stated on the printed insert that comes with an HIV ELISA Antibody test. In fact I was never shown that printed insert.

5)I was not informed that the proteins used in any HIV Antibody test have never been proven to be unique or specific for the HIV virus, or that many of the proteins used in the test kits have been found to be associated with things other than HIV in the human body

And so on for another 20 reasons. Then you may denounce the particular health center or doctor to the proper Medical Association, or not take the drugs they prescribe, or not see the AIDS doctors again, or whatever.

Why isn't it the same for 'HIV-positive' pregnant women? I learnt all about this now. The "therapy" – the State says – is preventive because 'HIV' is considered infectuous. But where are the proofs that it is infectuous? At that point, they all look at you as if you were lunatic. It is not their job to find the proofs. The doctors apply the protocol scrupulously, the nurses follow the orders blindly, the father is considered unauthorized to decide for his baby, the mother as well. If the latter object, the Children's Prosecutor is called to make them accept the decision.

But we are talking about a drug which has the skull and crossbones emblem on the lab's bottle and which is proven to increase the chances of the child getting sick soon after birth. [44]

Maybe the State Prosecutor should undertake the case, as "X" suggested in an earlier mail:

> Giving out any kind of drugs, especially those that are given out compulsory even though known to be harmful, demands scientific justification. If that doesn't exist then, the whole medical act is illegal and could do bodily damage by taking diagnosis etc...

I was for a while hopeless, fearing we would be unable to stop this. The proposed legal solution made me feel better.

3. Return to society

However I would soon need to have doctors again in my life, especially if I gave birth to a child. Whom could I trust after all that happened to me?

With surprise I saw that others now had the same concerns, especially the doctor Angelos Sicilian, the engineer Manos Kazakopoulos, and the therapist "X", all unknown to me until recently, precious friends by now. They wanted to work out how all this had happened, despite us living in a state of law, so we wouldn't make the same mistakes again. One way or another, they offered their own written testimonies for the mosaic I had started to put together.

Dr. Angelos Sicilian first showed up on my website to apologise on behalf of all

---

44 "AZT: Unsafe at any Dose? AZT and prengant women and children", Alberta Reappraisal AIDS Society (June 30, 2008), http://aras.ab.ca/azt-perinatal.html

representatives of Medicine in this country:

> Maria, I am ashamed to say that I am a doctor and microbiologist and that I had never managed to pass the twilight of AIDS and see what happens from the other side, even though all the facts were obvious: because I knew that I had many times seen patients who had a very low number of lymphocytes when suffering from a simple infection; because I knew that many antibody tests have cross-reactions for many antigens. To make up for that weakness of mine I thought to send Scovill's documentary – the one that was sent to me some hours ago and which I have now seen three times in the row without having enough of it – to as many friends as possible so that they too would be illuminated on the huge hoax it so clearly reveals.

He didn't need to get more enthusiastic about shedding more light on the subject; he believed that there is a route that leads to the truth. He wrote me a second message that would strengthen me forever:

> I believe that when you fight ignorance, you have to help both those who suffer from it and the few who keep the others in it. This war is inconceivable but it is real. What I mean to say is that you are like Neo – if you have seen Matrix – who was given the blue and the red pills. You chose the red one. You entered the real world of misinformation and illusion. You did not only enter it, but also managed to boot the Matrix (in the Greek version) so solidly that I am surprised to see the earthquake you caused reaches to the very feet of Gallo. It makes me wonder if you are the chosen one? The rest of us who took the red pill were weak and powerless to fight the Matrix. I wonder if we expected something like this would help us recover from our fear and our weakness. I really wonder what the next step is. I want to act as intelligently as possible, so I will now try to calm myself down.

We met at Angelos' office, drank tea and coffee, chatted like good old friends. He and Gilles found they had many points in common that they must be of the same age. We talked about medical treatments and wondered what was originally homeopathy's stand on AIDS? The answer came from Angelos Sicilian:

> "Vithoulkas had produced a study that claims HIV was produced in Los Angeles inside the bodies of homosexuals because they were taking a lot of antibiotics. In my opinion, he discovered only half of the issue. If he said that they didn't suffer from a particular illness and focused only on the weakness of the immune system, then he would be 100% correct. The first cases were all diagnosed with Pneumocystis carinii pneumonia. But, as the New York Times' article stated, not only did they have this but also a lot of other germs, viruses and fungi.

There can't be pneumocystis carinii pneumonia alone, as the writer of the article correctly notes. Its presence signifies a crushed immune system. The medical foolishness – I hope not dishonesty- was that there was no research into the medical history of these people to find the cause of their weakness. In Scovill's documentary (*The other side of AIDS*) it becomes very clear from the stories of the surviving homosexuals what had caused their weakness. The inhalants (poppers) and other drugs. This means that we owe an award to our great Vithoulkas who was the first one to make this public."

I had not known that Vithoulkas was honored in 1996 with a Right Livelihood Award, also known as Alternative Nobel Prize, for "working on practical and exemplary solutions to the most urgent challenges facing the world today." In Vithoulkas' case, "...for his outstanding contribution to the revival of homeopathic knowledge and the training of homeopaths to the highest standards." In Greece homeopathic training is only offered to medical professionals.

Another online acquaintance revealed the strength of this case. Manos Kazakopoulos, former engineer, cosmopolitan, wise, made the following introduction:

> Madam,
> I do not know if I am HIV-positive, nor do I care. My only concern is not to be immunosuppressed. Currently I suffer from an initial infection of Herpes Shingles. I take a 'toxic' drug, Valtrex, and every week I have to do liver tests. Of course, very few patients are subjected to liver tests because they take Valtrex. From what I understand, this special care is because I have ... medical "resorts" (jack as they say).
> The Valtrex monograph makes several points about the treatment of immuno-suppressed patients and the administration of this antiviral drug. I was upset when I read it! .. If indeed.? .. You helped me come round! Who? Me.
> Who am I?
> I have been a mechanical engineer for 42 years. I worked (in the early years) with the Smithsonian Institution (Astrophysical Observatory of Athens of the Greek National Polytechnic) and as the topography chair of this Polytechnic. Afterwards I left for Canada, where I was accepted in the Ordre des Ingénieurs du Québec. I dealt with research into the static strength of ice at the North Pole.
> About 10 years ago, I found in a basket of 'opportunities' at a large bookstore, the book "*Rethinking AIDS*" by an obviously ostracised immunologist named Bernstein. [45] I read it all (despite the medical

---

45 Robert Root-Bernstein, Rethinking AIDS, The tragic cost of premature consensus,

jargon) and I was so impressed that I made a presentation on the book at a club (Club de Lecture) where I was member. I had read all that was known at that time, including the facts Dr. Maniotis presented in his interview. My presentation raised many eyebrows, but not all.

As you may have understood, my hobby is medicine and I spent endless hours in study. But I live (we live) in a world full of idiots, who crucify those who carry inside them the curse of thinking. Now I'm no longer afraid of the Gerolymatos and Giannakopoulos of Vianex Inc.[46] because I'm foreigner and retired.

Still, you should be careful, for they will crucify you and the world will say…

Again, gypsies made the nails!...

Kavo Papas, (real name) Manos Kazakopoulos

An outstanding viewpoint, but what did the new supporter mean with his final quote from a song of Kostas Xatzis?[47] 'Ten truths if you say, ten times you will be crucified. And then, and then the world will say again. Gypsies, gypsies made the nails…' I wished he would explain it to me thoroughly some time, and that exactly happened the following week. He lived in Ikaria[48] but he would be in Athens for a few days so we could meet. He wanted to bring me the book that had impressed him, *"Rethinking AIDS. The tragic cost of premature consensus"* by Robert-Root Bernstein, a five-hundred-pages volume. We met during a chilly evening at the Esperia Palace Hotel, myself with Gilles, and Manos with his wife Marina. My new ally was like Sean Connery in his 70s. They had come with a motorcycle. We began with the book of 1993; noting how similar were its revelations to those that we were making today; and how vain it is to mess with such a finely made biological system. Bernstein said that, among the other paradoxes, we have patients with serious immune system damage that do not have HIV or AIDS, and healthy people with the HIV virus. This explains the weird wording of the message from Mr. Kazakopoulos: 'I don't care if I'm HIV-positive, my only concern is not to be immuno-suppressed.'

Many more people now seemed to be worried about their doctors' attitudes, as was also revealed on the website www.therapeia.gr/epilogi/. It stated: 'The Association for the Right to Therapeutic Treatment Choice invites all those who choose the alternative methods for disease prevention and recovery of health to become members of the Association and to support its efforts to guarantee the right of the Greek citizen to select his own therapeutic treatment.' The link was sent to me by Dr. Sicilian.

But when you realize what happens in AIDS cases and what is the reason for

---

Free Press, 1993

46 Vianex Inc., Greek pharmaceutical company

47 Kostas Xatzis (1936 -), Greek troubadour of the human rights

48 Ikaria, island of the Eastern Aegean Sea & the home of the mythical Ikaros.

your suffering all those years, how can you deal with your feelings about such a huge lie and continue with life? Gilles felt my anxiety, and said:

> "It is not enough to replace the AIDS doctors with other doctors and treatments. You will cure yourself alone. The biggest change is taking place inside you by transforming your awareness of things. This procedure has been described. It is called expansion of consciousness, you learn to see the world with brand new eyes.
>
> You have already done the first steps of this procedure, it was when you opened your eyes, a personal change usually caused by an external event or sudden flash that reverses all the familiar scenery. Then, you had to get free of the witchcraft inflicted on you and so gain a completely different sense of yourself; just like waking up from hypnosis and discoveing the existence of a different way of being that you couldn't see before. Afterwards, for a while you observe what was going on around you with silence and isolation, even though our age isn't in favour of periods of silence and immobility.
>
> You re-discovered the nature around you. It became much more intense when you started observing the trees, the water, the sun and the sky with new eyes. You embodied this new, personal experience of yours in sharing life with others, since you were always sharing values and beliefs. Finally, it was very important that you manifested this new vision of yours since you have gained it through a long period of preparation. But, unless you apply it in everyday life, it will remain an empty shell. You are now ready to heal; your organism will cure its wounds alone."

These steps towards a deeper vision of life are edited from the "Living Deeply" program of the Institute of Noetic Science[49], which has the slogan "Perhaps the only limits to the human mind are those we believe in" – from Willis Harman. Soon leaflets of the Institute were arriving addressed to myself. "Why are they sending them to me?" I wondered. "We are already members," said my beloved.

That morning, Gilles laid two printed pages from the Internet next to his hot chocolate. We usually have our breakfast around 7.00 am ." I have a gift for you today" he said. "Oh, yes, what?" I looked around. "Read this, " he said and showed me the pages. I did not hurry at all. After coffee, mini cheese-pies, a juice and my vitamins, I picked up the article: "The way of the Magician."[50] I

---

49 Institute of Noetic Science, dedicated to expanding science beyond conventional paradigms. Founded by Edgar Mitchell, the astronaut.

50 Jon Rappoport, The Way of the Magician, released to the No More Fake News Archives 2008-04-24.
   http://nomorefakenews.com/archives/archiveview.php?key=3393, last accessed February 8, 2009.

looked at it reluctantly. "Wherever the word "magician" appears, put instead the word "visionary," Gilles told me and walked off. I began to read:

Carlos Castaneda once wrote that a warrior takes everything as a challenge, while the ordinary person takes everything as either a blessing or a curse. This has a bearing on becoming a magician. If a person is dreaming up ways "to be blessed" all the time and takes no action, he will stagnate.

The magician rejects everything that comes out of consensus reality. He rejects it with greater power as he progresses. This rejection doesn't stifle him. It adds to his own creative power.

The magician isn't worried about how to fit in. He is already outside. What he creates has influence on the consensus, but that is not his aim. He is not in a constant state of grief about the condition of the world. He is not seeking to heal the whole world. For one thing, there are billions of people who refuse healing. That is their choice.

The magician sees that the very act of consensus---the very act of fitting in with the herd---is a surrender of self. Therefore, by definition, the consensus reality is going to be ill.

Nevertheless, the magician is willing to help---in certain situations, where individuals want to gain greater power.

The magician will also try to alleviate suffering when he sees an opportunity in certain situations, but this is not his constant aim.

The magician goes his own way. He builds and creates his own reality. That reality is unique to him. It is not a copy of some other reality. It is not a reflection of some system.

The magician is not seeking to align himself with some traditional way of "enlightenment." All such ways are tailored to fit the herd.

The magician is constantly creating. That is his energy and his place and his fortress. That is his challenge.

The magician does not need to be understood in conventional terms.

The magician is not trying to attain success by pleasing others.

The magician does not measure himself by conventional standards.

The magician is familiar with life. He is not naïve. He is not living in sterile isolation. He is not driven into a state of weakness and confusion by life.

The magician recognizes that societies are constantly preaching about "the common good" of the Group. He sees all that nonsense and he understands it is a form of surrender of the self. He sees behind the mask. He knows that many people are creating personalities for themselves based on that surrender. He understands that a true society would find ways to encourage the expansion of the self.

The magician finds his own road by creating it.

He is not looking for external concepts to which he can attach himself.

The magician surpasses every spiritual system and religion. These systems were built as a pale reflection of what magicians actually do.

I turned around to look at my man, to kiss him, to ask him once more: "How do you always know what I need before I even ask for it?" His eyes, the color of the sky, glinted. He proudly said: "Do you know what nickname I chose when I first went on Internet? Panoramix!" OK – but how my beloved know where to find my gift? Intuition. I now looked at the signature of the visionary, it was John Rappoport. Oh, it was the author of the book *"AIDS Inc, Scandal of the century"* that I mentioned earlier. And he wrote this new article on September 9th 2007, that is yesterday, just in time for me.

Certainly there are many categories of people in our society who will never react, because they are so focused on their personal benefits. However, opposite the pseudo wizards and their propaganda, there are always the visionaries, the real magicians. The "HIV-positive" ones, who have nothing to lose, could ally themselves with them. I suspected in this game of hunter and hunted the roles could be reversed at any time.

Chapter 7

Freedom: How I regained control of my life

1. Reactions inside Greece

While I hadn't announced from the beginning that I had stopped the AIDS pills, and delayed putting it in my website, I was suddenly looking forward to screaming it to everyone. Just in time, I got a call from the vibrant reporter, Christina Oikonomidou, who suggested that I participate the following week in the Vasilis Vassilikos[51] TV program "Axion Esti" about book writers. I had said that I would never go out on television again and I recalled Gilles telling me "Never say never." Truly, I didn't now even think about it twice. "Thank you very much," I answered melodically. "Shooting is scheduled this Monday." It was Tuesday, almost in a week. I would now give my whole being to preparing this interview. The show director was Takis Papagiannidis, we had the same family name by coincidence. We met each other for the first time and were sincerely glad. The interview would be aired on the ET3 state channel sometime soon. I spent the whole following week in high spirits gained from having this interview.

A few days later, I was presented with another challenge. '"X."' advised me to send an open letter to the Hellenic Association for the Study and Control of AIDS. It should be addressed to Mr Gargalianos-Kakolyris and Mr Lazanas, respectively president and secretary of this association. In my letter I should ask them to show us a photograph of the HIV virus and the proof that they claimed to have of its pathogenic action.

What a great idea of 'Mr "X."' again! One more time he would show me the way. I sent him an immediate letter and expected his reply by e-mail. He answered me the same day:

> You shouldn't just ask for the photograph of the virus. They have many of those and all are fake. Even if one photo were real, it would not be sufficient, the photograph must come with full description of its origin, so that we can confirm it. And of course, this is not enough either. We also need the proof that the particles shown are really what

---

51 Vassilis Vassilikos (1934 -), a prolific Greek writer and diplomat. His best known work is the political novel *Z* (1967), which has been translated into thirty-two languages.

they say, with their biochemical characterization and isolation from other particles. Unless there is a biochemical characterization, there can't be a vaccine to fight it.

Something like this would be enough, and so I wrote:

To Mr P. Gargalianos-Kakolyris, president of Hellenic Association for the Study and Control of AIDS, and M.K. Lazanas, secretary of Hellenic Association for the Study and Control of AIDS.
1/11/2007
Dear gentlemen,
As the new World Day against AIDS is drawing near, I invite you to take a step together in this direction.
Replying to your letter on behalf of the Hellenic Company of study and control of AIDS, sent 14/02/2007, in which you claim that my thoughts are extremely dangerous for the public health, that the HIV virus was isolated and photographed, and also that "there are irrefutable evidence proving that HIV causes AIDS", I ask you to present the proofs.
I am asking you to inform us when and where was the scientific paper published, according to which the existence of HIV was proven, and to present us this document so that we can verify its validity.
Additionally, we will also need the document that prove its pathogenic action.
Looking forward for your reply,
Maria Papagiannidou
maria@hivwave.gr

Naturally I would forward their answer, if it came, to Dr Andrew Maniotis who could spot their weaknesses. I included the letter in the introduction of my web page and expected it to bear fruit. They would be forced to send me the publications I was asking for, and either they would silence me forever or I would silence them. The letter was sent to the Hellenic Association for Study and Control of AIDS and to all medical reporters of the media in our country. The request was public, they ought to answer it.

But the Hellenic Association for Study and Control of AIDS completely ignored it and only took care to fill the electric trains and the subway with red posters and the motto "Don't catch...", printed on a sketchy plan of a condom with the words "Love, Life, Condom" on it like a garland. The same thing again. Like we should all live our life in fear of sex. I ran into this depressing poster on my way from Pallini. It was on the suburban railway, the subway and the bus. For a long time I could not avoid running into these ads that showed the signature of this Hellenic Association placed under a condom.

Entering my house, my first move was to delightedly open my favourite laptop, to enter my private paradise. I went quickly through the interviews I had given that were now up on my website. Each of them was then for me a kind of psychotherapy. I was being helped through answering questions. I particularly reviewed the points made by the journalist Varvara Georgiadou during an interview for the Cyprian magazine "Madame Figaro" for the World Day against AIDS .

I was impressed by the staff of this magazine, by their courtesy, their politeness, their tact. But when such people asked about my story, something had held me back. It was as though I didn't want to scare them so instinctively presented everything as rosy. To the question: "How did your family react? Were they panicked?" I responded: "Panic, no. When they found it out, when I was admitted to the hospital for the second time, they once again hugged me. In such cases, we support each other. Luckily for me they know how to support. They haven't changed their attitude towards me." Truly, but no one then knew what the other was doing in private. We were all crying. To the question: "How did your friends face it?", I had answered: "Likewise. It's not just a matter of friendship and love but also of spiritual composition. AIDS was and still is a cryptogram. It challenges you to solve it. My friends could only watch with interest what was happening to me." This was true, but their company couldn't console me much. I knew that their intentions were good, but I felt heavy as a rock. To the question: "When you said: 'Many times they thought they had lost me. You just expect to die,' what were you thinking at that time?" I had answered: "It wasn't so awful. Not for me. I only thought how this would affect my family. But I imagine they were used to the idea." I knew they weren't. They could never become so. I had embittered them for a lifetime. Then to the question: "Were you afraid of death?" I gave them the only absolutely true answer: "I guess I exorcised it. I reached the so-called near-death experience once or twice. And it was a nice feeling. Not pain, no problems, nothing. Just being peaceful, in empty space and ample light, moving forward. I had gone. Returning to reality displeased me. Mostly when my doctors told me, "You can live much longer". Should I be pleased? That way, I would be condemned to suffer hopelessly for much longer.

I remembered a related incident in Dostoevsky's *The Idiot*, in which the hero Myshkin tells of his encounter with a person being led to the firing-squad. "…They had already told him of his death sentence because of a political crime. Twenty minutes later they also told him of the decision on the reprieve. In the meantime, between the two decisions, he spent at least fifteen minutes of absolute awareness that he would die any minute. The last five minutes seemed to him like an endless deadline. He made a plan for the time he had left. He estimated the time needed to say goodbye to his friends: two minutes. Then, another two minutes to think for the last time about himself and one final minute to take a look around him for one last time. But nothing was more difficult to him than his obsession: What would happen, if he wouldn't die, if he regained life. What an eternity! Everything would belong to him, he would expand every moment to a whole century, he wouldn't miss anything, he wouldn't waste a thing!"

Oh, yes, I was experiencing that right now, no matter what others did. Triantafyllos of Salonika called and told me he was in Athens. He would go to the 19th Pan-Hellenic Conference of the Hellenic Association for the Study and Control of AIDS at the Caravel hotel. "Why don't you come for a walk, we can also chat a little" he suggested, as I had suspected he would. So, the 'pals' are having their annual conference. It was a sunny Friday, November 23rd, a week before the World Day against AIDS. The Caravel was nearby, but I wasn't excited about the idea. It would be just a waste of time. "Come, we can see new people, find other HIV-positives and see what they do with their medication." As Gilles was also enthusiastic, we decided to go.

The truth is that I had never been to an AIDS conference before and it was a good chance to take a look. I started smiling faintly as soon as we came closer, noticing its peculiar aura from a distance.

The entrance of Caravel was blocked by the parked luxurious cars of the guests, but no crowd. We entered the familiar neutral foyer, got to the lower floor and then witnessed the magnificence of the conference. It was like we had entered Hondos Center[52] in Pangrati. The products of the pharmaceutical companies were presented in fancy kiosks along with big posters of many young Adonises lying under the sun, with captions such as "Life goes on" or even without captions – the pictures were talking on their own. Yellow bags filled with gifts were distributed to doctors only. And many big names all around: Gilead, GlaxoSmithKline, Abbott, Boehringer Ingelheim, Bristol-Myers Squibb, Pfizer, Roche, Tibotec, Prezista, all the competing companies. Such a feast. Elegant employees stood behind the kiosks, ready to welcome us.

There were only a few people walking about. They had a cosmopolitan air, completely attuned to the presence of the security employees. The kiosk of the Non-Governmental Organizations looked like an exotic bird. I thought that there was no HIV-positives around until I saw my friend, Alexandra Athinaiou. That made sense as we were both authors of related books.

In the evening there would be a reception provided by the noble donations of big pharmaceutical companies. I surely didn't want to see that, but Gilles took my mom for the evening session. They wanted to listen to a speech about cases of HIV-positives who had stopped the AIDS treatment and restarted it. They informed me later that the scientists at the meeting only compared the number of the T-cells before and after stopping the medication. But they didn't speak at all about how people felt before and after. "We don't know the number of Maria's T-cells, as Maniotis told us not to check it", said my mom troubled. "Do YOU know the number of your T4? Do I? Why should Maria know?" Gilles told her with his sweetest manner.

Later the same day, my beloved showed me another news[53] item. "The Central Archaeological Council turned down a Health Ministry request for the Parthenon to be bathed in red light to mark World AIDS Day on December 1." Luckily, the Central Archaeological Council got in their way; it was a narrow

---

52 Hondos Centre, A famous cosmetics chain-stores in Greece
53 Kathimerini, 23/11/2007.
    http://www.ekathimerini.com/4dcgi/_w_articles_politics_1_23/11/2007_90420

escape.

Just as if he sensed what was coming, Vasilis Vasilikos decided to intervene and presented his Axion Esti TV program the following day, one week before the World AIDS Day. Finally, someone would throw cold water on them. Indeed, my appearance was a "living proof" that you can survive well without the use of AIDS medicine, even if you were nearly wiped out by their earlier usage. This made a great impression.

The reactions to my revelations were many and touching. It was alike what happened during the Olympics; people didn't just go for the victory but to participate. Let me start with a letter from that new HIV-positive friend from Crete. She is already present in this book, but was pseudonymous up until now:

> Good morning my dearest Maria,
>
> The reason for this letter was the tele-Marathon held today by ET1 (Greek national TV channel) about UNICEF with the subject "Child-Poverty-AIDS". Since they destroyed Africa by creating poor, orphan and sick children, they exploit the people's compassion and benevolence by organizing tele-marathons to gather money to supposedly "help" them. They are based on a hypnotized world which swallows everything they give it (THEY have hypnotized it, see USA).
>
> So I've changed my mind. I want you to write my name FULLY (FIRST NAME + SURNAME). So many people come out and state their opposition against AIDS. This way I am stating my opposition against the LIE of AIDS.
>
> Kisses,
> Ioanna

Did you understand who she was? The nicknamed Eleni, who had gone to Heraklio and found out that we are secret numbers like the prisoners of Auschwitz. Now she reclaimed her identity, Ioanna Dramitinos from Rethymno.

Another one warned me:

> Do not think that doctors were not in on it. You must not be fooled. When I asked a friendly doctor four years ago what to do because my condom broke while having sex with a girl, he answered "When I emigrate to Albania is when you'll catch the Aids virus...". Do you know how many cruises abroad he has been on!!!! Definitely over 28. There is no country or state. We are one big mess. They have panicked. They are losing the game. After Minnesota, there will be other states. And you know why? Because the pharmaceutical companies don't get along with each other and with the corresponding ministries.

Another voice: a 20-year-old youth who saw his friends dying.

Maria , they are stealing our lives...

I would like to help to make it possible to end this hypocrisy and mistreatment. Where are human rights? Every pharmaceutical company used us for their tests and led us to death... where is the UN to defend all the HIV seropositive victims? They are selling us off and we are just sitting down, letting it happen, killing us, torturing us, destroying us. All we ask for is deliverance and all they do is kill us. Who gave them the right to kill us? Does everything have to have a price? I am 20 years old and I cannot stand this rotten filth around us. Today one of my friends found out he has AIDS. Tomorrow it might be me. What should I do? How am I supposed to stand on my two feet when everyone ignores me? How Is possible that in 1984 people could enjoy sex at any time or place and nowadays they are sexophobic? What is the crime? Two years ago I was in London and saw people suffer, hurt, have really bad diarrhea, high temperatures and the drugs made them worse each day. And why all this? Who is going to pay for killing my friend Claudius at the age of 23? Who is going to pay for Sabina? AZT made her into a skinny miniature baby. I am sorry, we do not deserve this. It is not fair.

The father of a child unfairly lost:

Reversal! Earthquake! Dissolution of the mist! Rising light! Clearly visible target! May you and your companion be always well! And the "HIV-positives" who follow your route too so they mark it for all the others to follow. Unfortunately it's too late for me. Four years ago I lost my son (23). He belonged to the group of the "infected from blood products". He was diagnosed as HIV-positive many years ago, with... a 6-years-retrospective effect.(!) Through your web page and its references I analytically saw his whole story of the last 10-15 years. It was indeed that of a martyr, with all the anti-retroviral medicines and the infections caused by them. Eventually he "left" due to liver failure, like most have recently, as reported by specialists on your web page, but liver failure is not a typical AIDS illness. It's funny but I feel calmer now, for I found answers to my merciless questions. However, I am driven mad by the unfairness of this case, just like all the other cases. Experts are increasingly questioning the HIV tests and whether that virus causes AIDS. Our doctors who work in country of Hippocrates only care about advancing their career and prestige. The responsibility is huge. So the target is clear, let us all try to approach it, whatever this involves. Friendly.

A young homosexual man who was supposed to start his life when AIDS appeared:
... with all the commotion about AIDS that I have been hearing since childhood, I have suffered for the last 8 years from sex-phobia. Of course I am seeing a psychologist. I have been trying to enjoy life

and think I have mostly managed well apart from sexual contact. Not being able to be myself, I feel I am not complete and not free to use my own body. I have only been in contact a few times, because I could not relax and enjoy it. Every time I get suspicious, scared, and fear about the condom breaking and catching AIDS. And every 3 months I go off and get tested. I live a life of hell. According to science, being homosexual puts me in greater danger of catching AIDS. This is not a life, this is a decline of life. I intend to read the whole of your web page, I am already relieved. I hope to meet you. From the depth of my heart I owe you a big thank you and I am glad that I heard about you. I have a reason to live and not to medicate

An HIV-positive fellow who also took the decision to stop the HIV drugs after he read my story, said that there was also a 'Greek Duesberg' lady doctor! I did not know about that part of the AIDS history in our country:

I was found HIV-positive in 1989 and had the good luck to be under the care of Dr. Lianou, at the Report Centre in the University of Athens at that time. She was the only doctor (because a researcher) who would say that AIDS does not exist, it is immunodeficiency cases that we treat. She treated them with mega-doses of vitamin C!!!

As you can understand, after some years that Report Centre was closed by the professional unionists of HIV and I lost contact with the other guys. Any way, the cases she had treated were very severe, i.e. psychopath under therapy or junkies under drug use, and you know how both cases melt the immunodeficiency system. Yet I can let you know that they became all HEALTHY.

My mistake was that – after I broke up from a relationship that lasted four years, I fell into depression and developed an herpes zoster due to the immunodeficiency decay that followed. I went to the Syggrou hospital! There I was given the well-known treatments: that is herpes therapy plus HIV therapy: seemingly because my immunodeficiency system had hit the 'red', as if anyone else with herpes zoster would be strong as a turbo! So I fell into the pitfall and was taking the HIV drugs non -stop until I came across your website.

I did a flash -back and looked again at what had happened. I saw how stupid I was to stop the therapy by Dr. Lianou and turn to the bloody-pills of HIV! Since starting them, I have a very hard time with various dermatological problems, and lately my elbows were swollen to the size of eggs.

Anyway, I quit the pills six days now and my elbows already seem to be better! And the ferruci-forris dysplasia which had afflicted me for years though I had taken many drugs, even interferon, to calm it down with no results, now has started to fade away! (...) Gregory

Another one, shocked at what he had escaped:

Dear Maria

First of all I should thank you for existing and supporting people like me with your fight. I was diagnosed HIV-positive almost two years ago. I was going to the "Kratiko" (Greek national hospital in Athens) – where the diagnostics were done every three months to see if my antibodies dropped and I needed reinforcement with medicine. I then got a terrible depression and went to "Syggrou" (another Greek hospital) for psychological "support" because I supposedly shouldn't speak to my friends. To be short, I could not bear it anymore and I recently told my family, who had seen you by good fortune on TV when you were given the prize, We read your books and saw your interview.

I could not imagine the magnitude of this massive crime that came so near to me. I decided never to go to the "Kratiko" for tests again. Instead, only a check-up, like all the healthy people, for my general health.

A young scientist sent this heretical message fully signed, risking her own career:

...I have PHD in Life Sciences and I am a researcher at a foreign university. I work daily at a laboratory researching molecular biology and genetics. I am no AIDS/HIV specialist and I can't form an opinion about whether HIV causes AIDS or not, but I want to remark that IT IS VERY EASY TO PRESENT FAKE LABORATORY RESULTS. We experience this fraud every day in the lab., when we try to reproduce published results from other research teams and can't.

RECENT STATISTICS PROVE THAT HALF OF THE SCIENTIFIC PROJECTS ARE WRONG! I believe that beneath the AIDS issue lies a big lie, not a mistake.

...I wouldn't want my surname to show, nor the Foundation I work for. In order to report specific researches, I must have the agreement of my supervising professor and that isn't possible.

For example, about three years ago in the department where I work, they discovered that the results of an important project were made up. This work was published in NATURE but nobody wrote to this top journal to report this.

I know that there are supervising scientists who believe that HIV doesn't cause AIDS (I've also seen documentaries with scientific facts), but I wonder about the post-graduate students who work at HIV/AIDS labs and find out that their results show the exact opposite [to what they are meant to show.] What do they do...? They probably need to fix some scientific publications if they want to become academics..."

I wish you'll always be well
XXX

And a male nurse, ideologist communist, uncommitted:

> Good morning,
> My name is Angelos Vasilakis and I'm 28 years old. I work as an assistant nurse at the Athens Home for the aged. I'm absolutely stunned by what I saw and read on the site. I've studied 2 years at the former Middle Technical Nursing School of the Hellenic Red Cross. I've studied nursing for a year (second grade of education) at the 10 TEE (Technical Professional Education) in Pangrati. Today, I am in my third year at the First Department of Nursing at the TEI (Foundation of Technical Education) in Athens. Damn, I don't want to swear! But yes, I will! Up until today, I haven't heard a word of what you say and write! Even in between brackets. Even with depreciation; that this is AIDS, but there is also…a contradiction. Even if they depreciated it, they should mention it. They OUGHT to mention it.
> I studied nursing for six whole years. At the technical school, I was rather an attentive student yet I haven't heard a word.
> I confess that at TEI I'm not wonderful at listening to my teachers for many reasons. But if something so important, as the things you describe, was said, upon my Soul, I would have learned it!!
> I don't mean to tire you. Here's my point:
> Yesterday (19/1) I was working an evening shift. At the end of my shift the guys from the night shift arrived to take over. One of the most remarkable colleagues I've met until today gave me a paper with your site's address, and all she said was that I would be stunned by reading it. She did not tell me what it said.
> This colleague is neither a nurse, nor an assistant nurse. She is no doctor and has nothing to do with studies in the medical field. She is a waiter-cleaning woman.
> On my way back from work, I bought the Sunday newspapers and after I've read them I went to the website.
> And I was stunned…
> My colleague was right. ABSOLUTELY RIGHT.
> Which is her speciality again…?
> SHE IS OPEN-MINDED!! OH YES!
> TO HELL WITH THE SPECIALITIES, THE DEGREES AND THE ANTI-DIALECTICAL SCIENCE OF THE **!!
> I'll search whatever you say. I'll search to see if you're wrong.
> What left me stunned weren't your arguments. I haven't had time to study them and I guess this will take long. What has shocked me was THE CONTRADICTION. THE UNKNOWN CONTRADICTION. THE BURIED CONTRADICTION. If I see you're wrong, I'll find you and hoot you, even if it won't matter a lot. Otherwise, if I see you're confirmed, this time I won't be left stunned…

P.S.1: If my dear "Rizospastis" (Greek communist newspaper), wasn't concerned with the issue, there must be a good explanation for it...ARE WE OR ARE WE NOT COMMUNISTS!! WE HAVE THE RIGHT TO REPLY[54]!!

P.S.2: I am (still...) not an HIV-positive. I'm not black. I'm not dark. I'm not homosexual. SO WHAT??! WE HAVE THE RIGHT TO REPLY!!

A translator who reacted as if she had just woken from a deep sleep:

Dear Maria, I entered your web page for the first time on Sunday 28/10/07, and then I also entered www.peaceandlove.ca of your beloved Gilles. Honestly, I couldn't believe my eyes, although what I read were much more documented and reasonable than the things they have planted in our head like divine law all these years. Propaganda and the terror of an invincible threat are very effective. We are full of fear, we consider ourselves responsible and mature by doing this AIDS test to find out what? Absolutely nothing? Maria keep walking unshakeable, keep translating these shocking articles and interviews, otherwise, if we leave ourselves to the stupidity of the fear and the unfair isolation of the people...we are lost!

Other astonished people had questions like this:

Many organizations (like Doctors without Borders, Action Aid etc) promote their work and campaigns against many diseases in Africa and first of all AIDS (it is a catchy illness, not like Typhoid fever and the rest), asking for a small-for-the-'petit bourgeois' contribution to supply the medication of a child for 3, 6, 12 months depending on the sum of money given. My question is, if it is going to be revealed – the way it seems to appear on the horizon- the theater played at our expense, all that money goes to the pockets of some others. Only God knows what they are going to do with them!

It was the week following World AIDS Day, when the most unexpected event of the year occured. For the first time in the Athenian press, a front-page article was published entitled "AIDS, a global scandal." It was an interview of Dr. Maniotis by our correspondent in Washington Lambros Papantoniou. Of course I knew about it beforehand, but we could not be sure of its publication until it happened. The weekly that published it was "*Paraskevi* +13[55]", the only newspaper that had reported my request to be supplied with the proof of the HIV/AIDS concept by the Hellenic Association for Study and Control of AIDS.

---

54 Slogan of the communist party in Greece: Λευτεριά στον αντίλογο!
55 "Παρασκευή + 13". 'Paraskevi' means Friday.

It had also reported its failure to answer. I called the editor of the newspaper *Spyros Sourmelidis* to congratulate and personally thank him, and he agreed to let us post that interview on my website, where it is always available for everyone.

However, none of the major media organisations   commented on it. Complete silence. But nobody could alter this new reality: a whole 32-pages insert with an interview by a professor teaching in the largest medical faculty of the United States (University of Illinois in Chicago) had been published in the Athenian press and was accessible to anybody with a few clicks on the Internet. Mr. Sourmelidis and his colleagues should be proud of that.

2. Reactions outside Greece

We translated into English my first TV interview since I stopped taking the medicines, made for the program *Axion Esti*. We posted it, subtitled, in 'Google Video', and then notified the organization "Reappraising AIDS" headed by David Crowe of Alberta, Canada, in order to let the rest of the world know. Soon, my message was multiplied, returned rephrased from other people who were sending me their cases of liberation, from Italy, Spain, Ireland, U.S.A.

Julie from Ireland wrote to tell me that she had been diagnosed with HIV in 1997, started treatment in 2005 and stopped it a year later, for it had unbearable side-effects, causing peripheral neuropathy and mental confusion. She felt she had suffered a lobotomy every morning until midday, and at night she had to get to sleep before 10 pm to avoid experiencing the serious side-effects of the central nervous system that could follow. "We can say nothing good about this treatment. It is frightening to think people are being medicated for life with such toxic regimens, when so little is really known about what the medication is treating, if anything. There is so much mistrust. Fear propaganda is at play – covering up the huge lack of factual evidence that exits for what we are told by doctors and media, community health workers and researchers. It is madness."

Joanne, 55 years old, from New York wrote to say she was admitted almost dead to hospital two years ago. She had been deteriorating for a year, her hair were falling out, she was losing weight and it was impossible for her to eat anything as a result of anxiety related to a family case. At the hospital they diagnosed a serious fungal infection, as well as pneumonia and low haematocrit. Then the duty doctor diagnosed AIDS for the first time and presented to her a list of choices, including AZT. She started the treatment after a lifetime of systematic yoga, vegetarianism, organic diet and food replenishments and not a single visit to conventional doctors.
"Everything I avoided my whole life, I had suddenly to put up with because I didn't know what else to do. I stayed on medicine for a year and stopped them in previous May. This was an incredibly liberating and joyful day for me."

Isabel, from Barcelona, wrote that the reason she stopped the medication three years ago was that she was tired of living like a zombie walking around hospitals, and had learnt about the existence of the "dissidents". A wonderful period of recovery followed. She then enjoyed a body without lipodystrophy, travelling around Europe, living in Berlin. She almost forgot about AIDS doctors and inhuman hospitals, and now feels like "normal person", free of the heavy weight on her back.

But Isabel also wanted to spread the message. She gathered, with the help of friends and supporters, money to produce a video documentary. Swedish producers based in Barcelona wanted to help finance them to make it good enought for TV. "Patrizia Monzani is the co-director, she comes from Italy. We met in Berlin in 2005 when, with the Spanish journalist, Ali Saturio, we put our project together. Patrizia and I come from the art business and we both studied cinema. The documentary tells the story of a woman (myself) that, after going through hell, finds that all her suffering is due to the greed of the pharma industry. I can tell you about the first years of AZT, when most of my friends died before reaching their 30th anniversary. In the film we meet people who explain how they came to realise the truth. We have interviewed Spanish doctors, sociologists, seropositives who have taked meds and others who don't, mothers, biochemists, journalist, etc... and we will also include Duesberg, the Perth Group, Mbeki, Maggiore, Shenton, Liam Scheff, etc. We want to tell our story. Our story is yours and that of 1.000.000 more..." They have been working in this project for three years, in August 2008 they would gather the interviews and start the montage, so they suggested me having an "auto-interview" and I agreed with pleasure.

Soon after I received a message from David Crowe, director of the Alberta Reappraising AIDS Society, about another new production that I might like to participate in: "Gary Null is going to be doing a video on censorship in HIV=AIDS medicine and science. If you or your career has suffered as a result of questioning the HIV=AIDS connection, whether through denial of grants, ostracism, denial of tenure, etc, Gary will be interested in interviewing you. The focus of the interview will not be on how you disagree with the traditional theory, but on the price you have paid for disagreeing." About this, I do not have so much to say, at least not so far. But we could plan presenting the documentary in Greece when ready, as I know not everybody was so lucky as me in our country. There was a teacher in Thessaloniki who risked to be fired arguing about a hair-raising video which was shown every year at schools, titled "All the truth about AIDS". The horror in all its majesty.

On December 14th, another hopeful message from Dr Maniotis arrived. He helped Audrey Serrano, who was treated for 'AIDS' without reason, to win her court case:

> Hello friends,
>
> We have probably won the first AIDS case in a court of law yesterday, with 3.7 million as an indemnity, the Serrano case. This is a very important decision that shows ... how unreasonable the HIV testing is and the treatment that follows. [56]

---

[56] see http://www.cbsnews.com/stories/2007/12/13/health/main3614167.shtml

You can easily understand what happened at the Serrano case: they gave her the cure of AIDS by mistake and so she developed AIDS.

Soon afterwards, Stefano from Italy showed up, another 'HIV-positive' rebel who was very pleased to make our acquaintance – and wrote to me:

> I want to ask you: since the virus wasn't tracked and the test was never essentially approved, why do they keep talking about falsely positive results? Is there any truly positive result?

That was my question too. I was positive at every test I did, was this true or false? Better, should that test ever be recommended for anybody?

3. The turn of Justice

It was time for me to examine it further. Lawyers may have every good reason to win a race, but judges could possibly be bought. "Aren't there any incorruptible judges?" I once asked a young lawyer, Rania Katsarou, who had visited my website. "For these kind of cases there are other ways of pressuring. They get a warning that they will lose their promotion and stay in the same position for years, get sidelined, and may be sent on holiday to think about it."

It reminded me of a recent court case[57] in Australia, with Robert Gallo as a star witness, where the judge presented his decision favoring the official viewpoint after taking an unexpected holiday. We do not know if he was pressured in a similar fashion.

In Germany, there have been many legal actions undertaken by citizens asking fundamental questions about AIDS. 'X.' had observed them closely and he presents here the knowledge gained from this experience. There, the leading figure is Dr. Stefan Lanka, a virologist, who in a recent interview said the obvious: "I am not the only one claiming that that the so-called virus of AIDS, the HIV, was never scientifically proved, and that it is considered proved due to a "consensus." The Federal Health Minister Ulla Schmidt responded on the 05.01.2004 to the Federal Member of Parliament Rudolf Kraus: "'HIV is certainly considered, based on the global scientific 'consensus,' as scientifically proven [to be the cause of AIDS]."

Since then, everyone posing questions in Germany such as "where is the virus?" are rejected a priori as supporters of a Dr. Lanka who spreads lies. But he and his friends are also organised: they set up the organisation Klein-Klein-Aktion Organisation and build the site http://www.klein-klein-aktion.html where they gathered all the incontestable evidence. They also provide us with appropriate arguments and legal formalities, for the time being in German and

---

57 Parenzee case, decision given in April 2007 by a judge of the Supreme Court of South Australia. http://garlan.org/Cases/Parenzee. Also, the analysis of this decision in *Fear of the Invisible* by Janine Roberts (Ch. Entitled 'Searching for Fragments.')

soon in English.

The German Ministry of Health has ceased to claim that any pathogenic virus can be directly detected, because for years the citizens have again and again posed the question to the federal health officials, where is the scientific evidence of the alleged pathogenic virus. And what was the solution? After a multitude of actions in the German Parliament, the Federal Ministry of Health shifted the responsibility to the Federal Ministry of Research, which has now officially undertaken to deliver the most ridiculous point, that the legally guaranteed freedom of science leaves no room for the state to question any scientific claim.

The peak of that action, for us also to exploit, was the official correspondence between Prof. Niemitz and the federal Ministry of Health. "X" himself translated it into Greek. Niemitz reports in this official correspondence, the "confession" of the Minister of Health, that the 'AIDS' virus has not been proved scientifically to cause AIDS:

> H.-U. Niemitz, Probstheidaer Str. 10, LEIPZIG
> Mister Federal Minister Jurgen Trittin
> Commissioner Federal Minister for BMfVEL,
> Alexanderplatz 6,10178 Berlin
> Mr. Minister,
> In mid-November I am planning to hold an open assembly on the scientific basis for the prognosis of the Avian Influenza pandemic. This assembly will take place in Berlin.
> I have been greatly concerned about the prediction of pandemics from the mid-80s, from the non-appearance of the expected epidemic of AIDS to the somehow fitting reference in Parliament to the question of whether the AIDS virus, called HIV, has been scientifically proven. The answer, shocking for me, was as follows:
> "According to information from the Federal Ministry of Health (BMG), the proof of HIV with the electronic microscope, in the plasma or the serum of patients, has not been achieved ... "

This "confession" by a Minister is absolutely unique. This confession is one on which others can base serious criminal charges (complicity in crime against humanity, genocide etc). It will probably eventually make the doctors gradually stop supporting antibiotics and vaccines, either out of humanity or out of fear of a complaint from a patient, as all doctors will gradually be informed and wake up from the brain-washing lethargy they have long suffered from. Everyone will eventually know of this tragedy that has cost the lives of more people than all the wars of humanity.

This letter of Niemitz provides a good answer to the repeated allegedly unshakeable argument "you have no evidence to support the theory of non-existence of the virus":

> You have charged that I adopted some 'theory of non-existence ....
> As a scientist (and you are a scientist, otherwise from where did you

get the doctorate?) I should make it clear to you that there can be no 'theory of non-existence' in the physical sciences. If there were, then we could not resolve any dispute over the non-existence of anything... We cannot prove the non-existence of something... Logically (and therefore scientifically), the only truth can be that he who claims the existence of something, has also to prove it. And in this case you are the one! Namely, the Ministry of Consumer Protection and the Federal Government.

I found other models for bringing lawsuits. All the documents came from German books and cases. Among others, there was in X.'s dossier a copy of the magazine *Third Eye* [58] that told how to petition the European court in the Hague for legal action against genocide and other crimes against humanity committed by pharmaceutical companies. This is what it said:

The first person who signed such a complaint was Dr Matthias Rath, born in Stuttgart, Germany in 1955. After obtaining his degree he worked as a doctor and researcher at the University Clinic in Hamburg and the German Heart Centre in Berlin. In 1987 he discovered the connection between the lack of vitamin C and a new – at that time – risk factor for cardiovascular disease, litoprotein a. Following this discovery he began to work in 1990 with the two times (and almost three times!) Nobel Prize winner Linus Pauling. He went to the US where he was appointed director of Research in the field of cardiovascular disease at the Linus Pauling Institute in Palo Alto, California. His cooperation with Linus Pauling led him to study the relationship between nutritional lack in vitamins and other micro-elements, and many more diseases such as hypertension, heart failure, circulatory problems associated with diabetes, various forms of cancer, osteoporosis, diseases related to malfunctions of the immune system or AIDS.

In this petition to sue were named: Firstly, as legal entities, the multinational pharmaceutical giants 1, 2, 3 ... and as individuals the directors and the members of their Boards. Secondly, members of "Lobbying" companies that have actively participated in promoting "the interests" of the multinational pharmaceutical cartel or received financial benefits from it. Thirdly, individual politicians, as well as international and national political organizations which, during further investigations, will be found to have participated in the perpetration of crimes or benefited financially from it. Fourthly, employees of the general health field who, during further investigation, are found to have been deliberately and systematically involved for their own benefit in the promotion of the interests of the pharmaceutical cartel during the commission of the reported crimes. Fifthly, employees and members of the media who, during further investigation, were found to have been similarly involved...

---

[58] Issue 116, September 2003

But this bold doctor failed in his legal action. They stopped the trial or led it into a deadlock... Perhaps because he was not himself injured and there wasn't a specific offence under consideration, perhaps because they attacked his "Dr Rath Health Foundation." It had promoted globally a new model of health, aiming more at prevention and less at treatment, based on natural therapies and improvement in nutrition. He was accused of being a speculator, while they themselves were charged as "responsible for the systematic undermining of health, the cause of intentional damage to health and the death of millions of people around the world, deliberately committed for the promotion of their economic interests and business work on human disease."

It is also worth mentioning his research claim that taking vitamins can help in a large number of diseases (on his website there is more information: www.dr-rath-foundation.org). He has warned for years that there is a plan, through the Codex Alimentarius, to impose gradually a ban on vitamins beyond the very small dosage officially recommended. In 2007, the Board of the Greek EOF (National Medicine Organization) called for the IMMEDIATE WITHDRAWAL of all foods supplements containing vitamin C in quantities larger than 135 mg!!! However, it didn't make it clear if we should also avoid eating many oranges a day in case we exceed the "dangerous" level of vitamin C that others prescribe to treat heart diseases.

A phrase that circulates globally seems to be true: murder is allowed -- treatment is prohibited. 'We now have nothing to prove, they must bear evidence of what they believe and impose illegally ... by law', "X commented at the end: "This case can be undertaken by a lawyer pro bono, which means that he will be paid with a percentage of the compensation he'll win. There are such lawyers abroad, but I don't know what happens in Greece." There is an opportunity to create this field here, if it doesn't already exist. "Do you have a trustworthy lawyer to ask?" "I do."

A new person of equal brilliance would now appear in the foreground, the lawyer Rania Katsarou, a young woman (34 years old) with two children. She had earlier declared by e-mail her intention to deal with the issue when needed, and now I invited her to participate in the search. Not doing anything since we don't have any money was excluded as a possibility. "In life, as in all legal claims. everything begins with the demand.

If you don't demand, nothing and nobody is given to you. You Maria, have done otherwise. You reclaimed your life, your existence and your happiness. You have already won on all fronts. Only one thing is missing. Justification."

Epilogue

It is early spring 2009, nearly two years since I stopped taking 'AIDS' pills, and I don't get sick, I don't suffer in the evenings, I don't get tired when I sit, I enjoy every moment with my beloved Gilles – as if nothing had ever happened to me. Maybe my body is still injured deep inside, but I have found myself again and that is what counts more. I acquired a new realization of everything, got in contact with nice people that I would never have met otherwise, set goals that would have been previously considered unrealistic.

I understand this knowledge could be painful for those who lost beloved ones from AIDS during all these years, and I hope they will also get furious. Every day, new people unwittingly throw themselves into the 'seropositivity' fire, a living hell. We are unaware. Because we are not at war, we think we aren't threatened. Wrong. We are in a state of siege. It is beyond the scope of this book to define who, or what, lies behind the artificial HIV threat. My experience as described in this book only shows that we should not worry about "HIV."

Although it is not pleasant to bring everything back in my mind, it is impossible for me to watch indifferently for the rest of my life the misery of other 'seropositives' – because I know what happens when hope disappears. Citizens everywhere, not just HIV-positives, have the right to know that they can be released from fear, guilt, and the incredible restraints on life-and-death decisions based on a groundless theory.

Most healthy people have decided that they are not meant to learn how it is to be unafraid of love, and many elders have already forgotten how it was like to be young and free. Soon, there could be no one left who remembers what it was like living without that mental barrier created in 1984.

Call me romantic, but I dream that this immorality will sometime end. I'll give an example of a possible solution. In South Africa, after apartheid, the "The Truth and Reconciliation Commission" was created, essentially a court where anyone who believed that he was a victim of violence could be heard, where those believed responsible could be called to testify, so there was a record of the silent and immoral actions of the apartheid government, so those responsible could admit their mistakes. The purpose of the court was primarily to reveal the truth and to help with the creation of a new peaceful coexistence for everyone in the country.

Until something similar happens for AIDS, I am not allowed to forget anything, it would be like taking part in the crime. We have to record what has happened from the beginning, for the 25 years of AIDS. My own case alone occupies 24 of them. And I remember very well what was before, intermediate and afterwards. Meanwhile, more than 2,500 professionals, doctors, journalists and scientists have supplied us with demolition materials. What prevents us from burning this cloudy scene to ashes?

We are not at all alone. I hope my testimony will help create many more who reclaim the life that belongs to all of us. Businessmen, teachers, lawyers, carpenters – and doctors, all will learn to say "Good bye AIDS".

Appendix

As this book was in the corrections stage, another came out in France: *Les combats de la vie. Mieux que guerir, prevenir,* that is *The battles of life. Better prevent than fight,* by Luc Montagnier, co-discoverer of the HIV virus.

Surprise! The author suggests that stress could be sufficient on its own to cause AIDS, without 'HIV'! Here is the reaction of the ex-president of *Rethinking AIDS Group*, Etienne de Harven. It was sent to Maniotis on March *31 2008, and then to* me:

> Dear Andy, and all members of the RA Board, and friends,
>
> Yes, an incredible book has just been published, in French, by Luc Montagnier, under the title of "*Les Combats de la vie*", JC Lattès, editor, 2008, Paris, readily available via Amazon.
>
> I finished reading it 2 days ago, and I am still in some kind of a state of shock....
>
> The book starts with 138 pages of typical Montagnier's classics, such as HIV is not the only cause, mycoplasma should be looked at more carefully, nanobacteria also...
>
> Then, an extensive review on oxidative stress, with repeated indications of its likely causal role in AIDS. I had heard Montagnier speaking on that during his presentation in December 2003 at the European Parliament, Brussels during which he never made the slightest reference to Eleni Papadopulos, who, unless one of you can prove me wrong, was in 1988 the first one to hypothesize a possible link between AIDS and oxidative stress. I then went to chat with Montagnier, when the official part of the debate was over, and told him how surprised I was that he had so strictly ignored referring to Eleni's early paper! Back home, in February 2004, I wrote a long letter to him, including Eleni's reference...
>
> Throughout ... he gives the strong impression of having a broad paternity on the oxidative stress hypothesis... (I remember so well my former chief, Emmanuel Farber, speaking about free radicals 40 years ago...!) Then, he turns into an expert nutritionist on anti-oxidants, with a large interest on herbal medicine such as fermented papaya extracts, and an interestingly open mind on alternative herbal medications – and with very snappy remarks on the hardly justified huge profits of Big Pharma !!
>
> But the shock is in the final pages, when he recognizes that: -

scientific congresses became "great masses", where great priests pronounce the dogma that shall be distributed to their "slave-collaborators",

   - denouncing the sacred ritual of absolute dogma, and a tendency to eliminate disturbing ideas,

   - denouncing the formations of "closed chapels" where innovative ideas are excluded,

   - denouncing the exclusion from the scientific community of those who dare to deviate from the orthodox paradigm,

   - denouncing the "scientific monotheism" as a true perversion of real science,

   - and stresses that there is no place left for those iconoclasts who dare to shake the dogma...

   Sure, we all agree on all these points!

   But to hear Montagnier saying this, WHILE HE IS HIGHLY RESPONSIBLE FOR ALL OF IT, is where I find it absolutely shocking!

   A hypocritical monument...

   Of course, when the HIV/AIDS dogma shall finally collapse, this will make it easy for him to say "I told you so....

   Hoping to have stimulated your curiosity on this frankly surprising piece of literature!!

   And with my best wishes to all of you in all your projects!

   Kind regards,

   Etienne.

BIBLIOGRAPHY

Robert Root- Bernstein, The tragic cost of premature consensus, The Free Press, New York, 1993

John Lauritsen, The AIDS war. Propaganda, Profiteering and Genocide from the Medical-Industrial Complex, Asklepios, New York, 1993

Robert E. Willner, Deadly Deception, The Proof That SEX and HIV Absolutely DO NOT CAUSE AIDS, Peltec Publishing Co., USA, 1994,

John Stauber & Sheldon Rampton, Toxic Sludge Is Good For You. Lies, Damn Lies and the Public Relations Industry, Common Courage Press, 1995

Elinor Burkett, The Gravest Show on Earth. America in the Age of AIDS, Picador USA, 1995

Peter Duesberg, Inventing the AIDS virus, forwarded by Nobel Laureate Kary Mullis, Regnery Publishing, Inc, Washington D.C, 1996

Steven Epstein, Impure Science. Aids, Activism and the Politics of Knowledge, University of California Press, 1996

Christine Maggiore, What if Everything you Thought you Knew about AIDS was Wrong?, The American Foundation for AIDS Alternatives, CA 1996, third edition 1997

Peter Duesberg/John Yiamouyiannis, AIDS, Michaels Verlag 1998

Jon Rappoport, AIDS Inc. Scandal of the Century, Truth Seeker Company UK
(first edition 1998), Namaste Company USA (second edition 2004)

David Allyn, Make love, not war. The Sexual Revolution: An Unfettered History, Little, Brown and Company, 2000

Michael Leitner, MYTHOS HIV, Verlag videel OHG, 2000

Steven Ransom & Phillip Day, World Without AIDS, Credence

Publications, England, 2000

Gary Null with James Feast, AIDS. A second opinion, Seven Stories Press, New York, 2002

John Crewdson, Science Fictions, A Scientific Mystery, a Massive Cover Up, and the Dark Legacy of Robert Gallo, Little Brown and Company, Boston, New York, London, 2002

John Stauber & Sheldon Rampton, Trust Us, We're the Experts! How Industry Manipulates Science and Gambles with your Future, Penguin, New York 2002

Gerhard Buchwald, Vaccination: A Business Based on Fear, translated into English by Erwin Alber, Books on Demand 2003.

Karl Krafeld/Stefan Lanka/u.a., Impfen – Völkermord im dritten Jahrtausend? klein-klein-verlag, 2003

Jean-Claude Roussez, SIDA, Supercherie scientifique et Arnaque humanitaire, Marco Pietteur, editeur, Belgique 2004.

Karl Krafeld/Stefan Lanka, Das Völkerstrafgesetzbuch verlangt die Überwindung der Schulmedizin!, klein-klein-verlag, 2004

Michelle Cochrane, When AIDS Began. San Francisco and the Making of an Epidemic, Routledge, New York and London, 2004

Etienne de Harven & Jean Claude Roussez, Les 10 plus gros mensonges sur le Sida, editions Dangles, France 2005

Celia Farber, Serious Adverse Events, An Uncensored History of AIDS, Melville House Publishing, 2006

Stephen Davis, Wrongful Death, The AIDS Trial, a Novel, Virtualbookworm.com Publishing Inc., 2006

Stefan Lanka/Hans-Ulrich Niemitz/Veronika Widmer/Karl Krafeld, Die Vogelgrippe – Der Krieg der USA gegen die Menschheit, klein-klein-verlag, 2006

Stephen Davis, Are you positive? Virtualbookworm.com, 2007

Rebecca Culshaw, Science Sold Out. Does HIV really cause AIDS?, foreward by Harvey Bialy, The Terra Nova Series, 2007

Henry H. Bauer, The Origin, Persistence and Failings of HIV/AIDS

Theory, McFarland & Company, Inc., Publishers, 2007

Torsten Engelbrecht & Claus Kohnlein, Virus Mania. How the Medical Industry Continually Invents Epidemics Making Billion-Dollar Profits At Our Expense (translated by German), Trafford Publishing, 2007

Luc Montagnier,Les Combats de la vie, JC Lattès,Paris, 2008,

G.Vythoulkas, A new dimension in Medicine, Adam ed, 1994, 1998

G. Vythoulkas, Homeopathy - Medicine for the new Millenium, Parisianos Scientific Publications, 2001

Janine Roberts, Fear of the Invisible: How scared should we be of viruses and vaccines, HIV and AIDS? Impact Investigative Media Productions, 2008. `New edition 2009.

Video Documentaries:

-HIV=AIDS, Fact or Fiction?, by Stephen Allen (1997)

-Deconstructing the Myth of AIDS, by Gary Null (2004)

-The Other Side of AIDS, by Robin Scovill (2004)

-Guinea Pig Kids, by Liam Scheff (2004)

-AIDS Inc., by Gary Null. (2007)

GLOSSARY

AIDS (Acquired Immune Deficiency Syndrome): The definition of AIDS differs from continent to continent, and even from country to country, and has changed a few times since its initial phrasing by the American CDC. According to the definition in effect today in USA and adopted in Greece as well, AIDS is not an illness but is – as its name shows – a syndrome of immune deficiency, that is a collection of more than 25 already known diseases which may also occur in people who had a HIV-positive reaction. The cause of AIDS is considered to be HIV retrovirus, though the syndrome initially appeared in people who abused heavy recreational drugs, and were taking plenty of antibiotics. AIDS may be diagnosed in anybody who has been found "HIV-positive," when they develop any one of these 25 or more illnesses. In other words, pneumonia to someone who was found HIV-negative is called pneumonia, while to someone who was found HIV-positive it is called AIDS. In the first case it is treated with the pneumonia antibiotics and is considered curable, in the second the person is given the pneumonia antibiotics together with the toxic life-long" AIDS therapy."

Antibody HIV tests: These tests are a non-transparent selective method which determines who will be named "HIV-positive" and consequently an "AIDS patient" afterwards.

HIV (Human Immunodeficiency Virus): The misleading name given to a retrovirus that allegedly causes 'AIDS'. The existence of that allegedly pathogenic virus has never been proven, so it is nothing more than a presumption that is promoted as a real fact. The electron microscope images presented since 1983 as a proof of the existence of HIV, only show normal cellular constituents and debris; none present a properly isolated virus with the necessary scientific documentation.

Isolation of a virus: Part of the process with which the existence of a virus is proven. It aims for the separation of individual viruses from any surrounding components and particles, so that the resulting electron microscope photographs show only uniform and equal-sized particles that have then been proved to cause the disease in question. This process has never been demonstrated for 'HIV".

The Gallo Papers: 4 scientific papers published in *Science* in May 1984 that were widely acclaimed to proving that HIV causes AIDS. It has since been established that a significant degree of scientific misconduct occured during these papers formulation, sufficient to cast very severe doubts as to their validity. This evidence led on December 4th 2008 to the *Science* journal being requested by over 30 scientists and medical doctors to have these papers withdrawn. At the time of going to print, this matter was not yet resolved.

Proof of a virus: Advanced process to demonstrate the existence of a virus. It requires isolation of the virus, photograph by electron microscope and biochemical characterization.

AZT: Medical drug developed in the '60s for cancer. Although it was considered too toxic for cancer patients, it was approved for AIDS on the basis of fraudulent clinical trials.

Retrovirus: A particle produced by the cells of animals, fish and plants, that carries a strand of RNA and enzymes within a protective envelope of proteins. Like most viruses, it is approximately a millioneth of the width of a cell and totally inert with no metabolism. When originally observed entering cells, it was assumed by many that they were pathogens, but we now know that, among other things, they are a means by which cells share genetic information and thus communicate. This process plays an important role in cellular evolution and apparently can assist cells to adapt to meet new dangers. Some retroviruses are also reported to have strong anti-tumour effects.

Anti-retroviral therapy: A form of chemotherapy, often using AZT, that is aimed at preventing cells from making retroviruses, as HIV is said to be a retrovirus. It is not targeted soley against HIV as the latter is said to be very hard to find in a patient. Its 'efficacy' is estimated with the invalid CD4 and viral load measurements. However, anti-retroviral therapy has been shown to increase morbidity and mortality of 'AIDS' patients, even with the latest medications.

CD4 tests: The CD4 tests measure the number of a specific type of white blood cells in the blood, and are used only for 'HIV-positive' people. They are considered critical in assessing the immune system of 'AIDS' patients, and the efficacy of the therapy. However, any acute illnesses, such as pneumonia, influenza, or herpes, can cause the CD4 count to decline temporarily; it has nothing to do with 'HIV'.

Viral load: The 'viral load' is estimated by a test which allegedly calculates the quantity of 'HIV' in the blood, using the PCR method that the Nobel Prize winner Kary Mullis developed although he himself said his method cannot measure the prescene of HIV.

Homeopathy: Therapeutic method and integrated medical system, developed in the late 18th century by the German physician Samuel Hahnemann. It is a pharmaceutical method, free from side-effects and based on specific laws.

AIDS "Orphans": In Africa 'orphan' means the absence of one parent, temporary or permanent. They may have died, or could be working or fighting far away, as the singer Madonna found out when she was introduced to her orphaned child's father.

The Author

Maria Papagiannidou Saint Pierre is a senior Greek journalist and an 'ex-AIDS' patient. She has lived as an anonymous HIV-positive person for almost her entire adulthood.

Born in January 1965 in Komotini in northern Greece, her parents were a philologist and a mathematician. With her family she moved to Athens when 5 years old. She read Greek Literature at the University of Athens and did postgraduate studies (Master in Classics) at the University of London. She was diagnosed "HIV positive" in 1985. In January 1989 she began writing for the newspaper "*Vima on Sunday.*" From 1995 to 2005 she was a full- blown AIDS patient. In January 2006 she started the website www.hivwave.gr as Maria K. to publish her reseach on AIDS. In May 2006 she published the book '*Maria K. How I defeated AIDS, a wonderful adventure with the HIV virus.*' (Kastaniotis publications) In July 2006 she married the Canadian biologist and computer technician Gilles Saint Pierre. Her second book was published in March 2007 and entitled "*The game of love at the time of AIDS*" (Kastaniotis publications), this time under her full name of Maria Papagiannidou Saint-Pierre. On 23 April 2007 she stopped taking the pills prescribed against AIDS, recovered her health and regained the freedom that we all lost in 1984.

Author's website (English/Greek) http://www.hivwave.gr/pages/en/

LaVergne, TN USA
29 September 2010
198863LV00006B/26/P